THE BODY OF THIS DEATH

Historicity and Sociality
in the Time of AIDS

The Body of This Death

HISTORICITY AND SOCIALITY
IN THE TIME OF AIDS

WILLIAM HAVER

STANFORD UNIVERSITY PRESS

Stanford, California

Stanford University Press
Stanford, California

© 1996 by the Board of Trustees
of the Leland Stanford Junior University

Printed in the United States of America

CIP data appear at the end of the book

Stanford University Press publications are
distributed exclusively by Stanford University
Press within the United States, Canada,
Mexico, and Central America; they are
distributed exclusively by
Cambridge University Press
throughout the rest of the world.

for Harry Harootunian

Acknowledgments

This book has benefited from comments from a number of people whom I am grateful to know as colleagues; even more has it benefited from discussions, differences, arguments, brawls, and even occasional agreements, with those same colleagues. I am particularly indebted for their support and colloquy to Bat-Ami Bar On, Judith Butler, John Chaffee, Brett de Bary, Marilyn Desmond, Paul Dottin, Sarah Elbert, Risa Faussette, James Fujii, Yukiko Hanawa, Gladys Jiménez-Muñoz, Gerald Kadish, J. Victor Koschmann, María Lugones, Alice Pitt, Ellen Radovič, Katherine Rudolph, Kelvin Santiago-Valles, Joan Scott, Israel Silva-Merced, Joseph Suglia, and Maureen Turim.

Cat Lam has been most helpful in her enthusiastic searches for materials on David Wojnarowicz; Ron Palmer's prose poems, in their unrepentant queer eroticism as well as in their formal virtuosity, heartened me at a critical juncture; Stephen Barber has courageously responded to my work from the only place where a judgment has any consequence whatsoever; Sue Golding, in her existential comportment, as in her work, has been nothing less than something like an inspiration; Michael Bresalier made writing on Wojnarowicz and Golding a difficult and painful process, for which I am sometimes grateful. Naoki Sakai and I have been talking, drinking, and arguing for years; in the instance of the present essay, I am especially indebted to him for discussions of Nishida, Ōta, and Tanizaki—and so I hereby forgive him for accusing me of Lacanianism. I thank Gary Wickham, erstwhile intellectual companion and lesbian-brother-in-residence, for doing all the cooking during the writing; and I thank Winston and Salem for their sovereign indifference to it all.

Deborah Britzman and Christopher Fynsk have been with this project since it was but an infant paragraph. It would be impossible to exaggerate the debt I owe to each; if I have even approached something that might be called thinking, it is because they have encouraged me to join them in the audacity of their intellectual insubordinations. This thing is as much their fault as it is mine.

When this book reaches print, it will be fifteen years since I met Harry Harootunian, mentor, colleague, and friend. What counts for me as the world would surely be a safer place had I not encountered him; just as surely, it would be insufferably dull. So, in dedicating this book to him, I merely mark the impossibility of any adequate acknowledgment of the gift of that friendship.

W.H.

Contents

Preface

Q. Why did the monkey fall out of the tree?
A. Because it was dead.

—David Wojnarowicz, *Close to the Knives*

Impossibly, but necessarily, the body of this death is at once singular and multiple. In both its singularity and its multiplicity, but above all in the essentially erotic conjunction of its singularity and multiplicity, the body of this death is an impossible object for any apperception, any phenomenological apprehension, any auto-affectivity, any specular capture. This book is therefore not about representations of the body, nor even about the "body" as a possible object for representation; rather, it is about that which is the occasion for any possible representation whatever. In other words, this book is written around that which it will necessarily always be impossible to say, the ultimately unspeakable radical historicity and sociality of erotic existentiality. Here, then, the "body of this death," the erotic body in its historicity and sociality, an unimaginable figure, designates the thought of that which it is ultimately impossible to think. A thought, therefore, of the limit, to be sure; but also, and as such, a thought of the ethico-political as something other than the mere actualization of a possibility.

The body of this death is singular precisely to the extent that it is the failure as such of any recuperation or redemption, precisely to the immeasurable extent that it exceeds the figure of the particular in any dialectic. The body of this death is the incommensurable singularity of the *ipse* in its materiality. Now, if this invocation of the materiality of the body of this death is to figure in thought as something other than an excuse for a certain transcendence, it must mark the radical nontranscendence of absolute separation as such. The body of this death, the unimaginable figure of zero-degree historicity, figures the very inescapability that is its existentiality. The body of this death, in and as its material existentiality, belongs to death. It is not merely that it is obliged to die in some universal *devotio*, in which case death would be merely the proleptic predicate of its being, but that it is situated (or "thrown") between the first death of that death sentence called birth, and the second death of annihilation, of nonappearance. Indeed, the body of this death *is* that situatedness, that situation itself, that historicity. Inescapability is therefore not merely a fate or destiny that befalls the body; rather, the material body *is* that inescapability, that nontranscendence, that destitution.

We cannot evade the fact, however distressing it may be for a thinking that seeks the comfortable consolations of its own transcendence, that this inescapable belonging to death is the object of an essentially disturbing affirmation for a number of figures. At the end of John Greyson's film *Zero Patience*, Patient Zero, refusing redemption within an orthohistoriographical practice, affirms the inescapability of the body of this death in singing, "Make me true, make me clear, make me disappear"; and then, in the fusion of fire and water at zero hour, in the disjunct simultaneity of contradiction at the very limit of thought, in the *ekstasis* of zero-degree temporality, Zero disappears.[1] Or again, very near the end of his life in 1992, David Wojnarowicz produced an untitled work, a photograph of bandaged hands, with a silk-screened text tattooed across the photographic image that reads, in part:

> Sometimes I come to hate people because they can't see where I am. I've gone empty, completely empty and all they see is the visual form; my arms and legs, my face, my height and posture, the sounds that come from my throat. But I'm fucking empty. The person I was just one year ago no longer exists; drifts spinning slowly into the ether way back there. I'm a xerox of my former self. I can't abstract my

own dying any longer. . . . I am crawling and looking for the aperture of complete and final emptiness. I am vibrating in isolation among you. I am screaming but it comes out like pieces of clear ice. I am signalling that the volume of all this is too high. I am waving. I am waving my hands. I am disappearing. I am disappearing but not fast enough.[2]

And was it not Michel Foucault who sought a writing "in which I can lose myself and appear at last to eyes that I will never have to meet again"? He continues, of course: "I am no doubt not the only one who writes in order to have no face. Do not ask who I am and do not ask me to remain the same: leave it to our bureaucrats and our police to see that our papers are in order. At least spare us their morality when we write."[3] In Greyson, Wojnarowicz, and Foucault, then, the affirmation (albeit "nonpositive") of the body of this death, in and as its incommensurable singularity, its materiality and historicity (its belonging to death), its inescapable destitution, *is* its irreducibility to sheer visibility or representability. It is in part the work of this text to think what the consequences of the irreducibility of the material body of this death to representation and hence to thought might be for representation and thought.

But my purpose in attempting to figure the inescapability and irreducibility of the body of this death is not in the first instance (and least of all in the last) to produce a new and improved historical Imaginary, or even the epistemological ground of such an Imaginary. Rather, in thinking the thought of a historicity that is irreducible to conceptuality, I attempt to begin to think the thought of an erotic sociality that would be the destitute being-in-common of whatever singularities, and hence the ethico-perverse: the political.

For the singular body of this death is simultaneously, and impossibly, multiple. The multiplicity of the body of this death must not be thought, however, to be the degeneration or fragmentation of a prior unity; this multiplicity must be thought to be originary. Here, therefore, the multiple cannot be construed as the simple opposite or negation of the singular; this is not the relation of the universal to the particular, in which the particular as such would be

merely the dispersion of the universal. Yet neither does the thought
of the multiplicity of the body of this death merely figure the entropic shambles of a hecatomb. Nor yet, if we are to think what
must be thought from within the specificity of the historical situation of the AIDS pandemic, is this simply the thought of the absolute empirical contingency of the "flux." First and last, any
thought of the originary multiplicity of the body of this death must
take up, as the most serious of its requirements, an attempt to think
the originary sociality of our being. A very large body of work has
persuasively argued that sociality, or relationality as such, logically
and existentially does not so much "precede" its articulations, but is
rather co-extensive with, and as, articulation altogether. If we are
serious here, it seems to me that we must therefore think sociality as
vulnerability, as anonymity, and as a certain erotic nomadism. It is
not, of course, that essence would precede existence, nor merely
that existence would precede essence, but, perhaps more radically,
that fucking precedes existence, rendering essence irrelevant. What
is at stake here is a certain existential promiscuity, the erotic nomadism of the stranger, the fuck-buddy. (And here I want to acknowledge that recent discussions with Sue Golding and Christopher Fynsk have contributed inordinately to these formulations.)
What is at stake here is the priority of a rendering oneself vulnerable to the risk of the stranger over any structure of intersubjective
recognition in the quite literal multiplicity of "the body" in orgias-
tic group sex, for example. What I want to pursue, in this and subsequent books, as well as in various other practices, is the possibility
that there is, theoretically and practically (supposing one were to
admit that differentiation), a coincidence of a destitute being-in-
common of whatever singularities with the vulnerable, anonymous
encounters of erotic nomads. This would constitute what counts as
disappearance in Greyson, Wojnarowicz, and Foucault, not as a sac-
rificial invisibility in a communitarian aesthetic sublime, but as an
aesthetic from within which, and as which, the figure of the ethico-
perverse might appear.

   To be sure, this book only approaches such a possibility in an
entirely tentative and largely inchoate fashion; in this sense, the en-

tire book is merely prefatory, for what is at stake is the possibility of a queer—perverse—erotics. If we are to think the conjunction of historicity and sociality, if we are to think the simultaneity of the singularity and multiplicity of the body of this death as something other than a banal nihilism, then we must think the necessary heteroclite conjugation of the perverse, the ethical, and the political. My argument in this book is that it is only in thinking the originary conjunction of the historico-social to be an erotic conjunction, in thinking the primordial coincidence of the singularity and multiplicity of the body of this death to be an erotic coincidence, that the figure of the ethico-political as such might emerge. And this movement—from the thought of a radical historicity, through a consideration of the essential vulnerability, anonymity, and nomadism of erotic sociality to that impossible site where the figure of the ethico-political might emerge—has required that I follow a perverse, queer, itinerary.

In "Not Even a God Can Save Us Now," I attempt to think, in relatively general terms, something of what might be at stake for any consequent thinking in the time of AIDS; it is an attempt to say, from within the specificity of our current historical situation, what might be at stake in the thought of nontranscendence, of historicity. The "First Excursus on the Divine Right of the Historian" proceeds, through a reading of certain extremely problematic texts by Nishida Kitarō, to attempt to mark the limit of a thinking (frequently characterized as "modern") that in its promise of various forms of transcendence occludes historicity as such. We are familiar with various forms of this modern aspiration to transcendence— liberalism, fascism, the dialectic, for example—which are certainly not the "same thing," but share a certain logic, and are thereby mutually complicit. In Chapters 3 and 4, I turn to a reading of texts written by Takenishi Hiroko and Ōta Yōko in the aftermath of the atomic bombings of Hiroshima and Nagasaki. I do so in order to specify something of the dimensions of what a consequential consideration of the historico-social might entail in a time when genocide is always a present possibility. In "Y Su Sangre Ya Viene Cantando," I turn to a consideration of erotic sociality in the time of

AIDS, specifically as articulated in texts by David Wojnarowicz. Central here are the themes of vulnerability, anonymity, the erotic, and nomadism. The "Second Excursus on the Divine Right of the Historian" turns to a reading of Tanizaki Jun'ichirō in order to consider the possibilities of and for historiographical representation as something other than the adequations of an unreflective mimesis, and consequently to consider the possibilities of the parodic as a fundamentally perverse, queer practice. Finally, in "The Death of Michel Foucault," I read selected essays by Sue Golding in order to think toward the necessary conjunction of the ethical, the political, and the perverse; in order, that is to say, to think toward a politics of inconsolable perversity.

Thus, this book that you have just begun to read you may well find to be irritatingly episodic, fragmentary, and eclectic, frustrating at once in its utter banality and in the obscurity of its allusiveness. The fragmentary, repetitive, banal, and obscure aspects of this book are, it seems to me, unavoidable effects of a continuing attempt to find a question worth asking—for once in our lives, anyway. For once in our lives, let us admit that most of the questions we ask, however profound they may be, are (no less profoundly) irrelevant to the brutal facticity of the lives we must live and the deaths that, at least once in our lives, we must die. No text, about AIDS or anything else, has ever saved a single life. This irrelevance is not in the first instance a matter of the bad faith, intellectual laziness, or sheer stupidity of those sociological objects called the academic or the intellectual (although you, as readily as I, will undoubtedly be able to think of examples of those who exhibit such attributes). Rather, this irrelevance is at once structural and essential. A structural irrelevance insofar as the entire force of our institutional and professional lives works to keep us from distinguishing between necessary and unnecessary compromises, to domesticate us in our disciplinary bondage, to keep us, as "concerned scholars" or "concerned faculty," from acting up, from any serious engagement with the existential demand of a world we profess to interpret, from the danger of what it might have been to think, from the risk of madness and death.

Our irrelevance is essential to the extent that our structural irrelevance is no accident, insofar as it is the institutional expression of
the occlusion, in and as thought, of the erotic, of historicity and
sociality, ultimately of the political. To the extent that thought is
not a thinking at the limit of what it is possible to think, to the extent that thought does not think itself to be a thinking up against the
wall, to the extent that thought assumes the possibility of thinking,
of language, of history and sense, thought necessarily thinks the
world as a place where thinking is possible, and thereby resigns itself
to metaphysics. Now this question of the limit of the thinkable has,
of course, been a central concern for a scant few of those who, regardless of their professional franchise, are called philosophers. My
only point here in invoking such august company is that the question of a question worth asking, that any attempt to think, for once
in our lives, toward a question worth asking, is necessarily fragmentary, repetitive, banal, and obscure. I say this neither as apology
for nor in justification of the scrappiness of this thing you are evi-
dently still reading, but to suggest that the question I want to ask,
which revolves around the aporetic thematics of "AIDS," "historicity," "sociality," "praxis," and "ethicality," may ultimately be a question it is impossible to pose, around which only fragmentary and
repetitive maneuvers—a guerrilla questioning (an intervention)—
is possible. Finally, let us admit that the only historical question is the
question of the historical, that the only social question is the question of the social, that the only ethico-political question is the question of the ethico-political. For once in our lives, finally.

Thus, I hope this thing you are reading will amount to a
polemic, by which I mean not only the refusal of every irenic discourse, and not only the truncation of the arguments that would
support specific statements, but also an attempt to intervene in a
specific situation. Here I take "intervention" to denote provisionally,
and perhaps provisionally at best, the relation of the essential diffi-
culty of thinking to the force of certain determinate exigencies, the
force of the existential, in this case of what is called AIDS. But by
polemical intervention I also mean that this intervention refuses to
participate in the contest to establish intellectual hegemony, to pro-

vide a more persuasive explanation of the world; this is therefore an attempt to contest the grounds of the so-called "conflict of interpretations." I attempt, however ineptly, to situate this intervention at the level of the inaugural epistemological gesture by which the aspiration to knowledge, whatever else it may posit, and *in* positing whatever else it may posit, posits its own possibility. I do so in the interest of what I think must still be called revolution, if for no other reason than the lack of a better term (a lack that is not accidental).

Let me say as clearly as I can that in what follows I mean to say that what is called AIDS poses an essential threat not only to our commonplace assumptions about the capacity to manage or control the pandemic, but also to our equally commonplace assumptions about the nature of the world, the social, the economic, and the political—and *thereby* to the assumption that it is possible to posit the world as an object of knowing. It is therefore necessary to recognize that any serious and *consequent* engagement with what is called AIDS will be possible, if at all, only in a radical questioning of what we take, by and large, too often to be the unproblematic ground of knowing. Such an engagement therefore demands an openness to the radical insecurity of a futurity for which we must refuse to be prepared, an openness to a revolution that would be at once political, economic, social, cultural, and intellectual. Such conceptual demarcations themselves, as well as the institutions they in the last instance sustain, will of course not withstand a serious engagement with the questions of AIDS.[4]

THE BODY OF THIS DEATH

Historicity and Sociality
in the Time of AIDS

CHAPTER I

Not Even a God Can Save Us Now

The Originary Multiplicity of the AIDS-Object

What is called AIDS is, for consciousness and for thought, a necessarily impossible object. As such, and in itself, AIDS is radically unthinkable, resisting objectification, interpretation, the understanding, meaning, and the aspiration to transcendental subjectivity absolutely; AIDS belongs to that to which every teratology, phenomenology, or hermeneutic is necessarily and forever inadequate. In this project I shall therefore not attempt to interpret and therefore understand AIDS, to think what is radically unthinkable. Rather, my project is to think the specific determinate unthinkability of what is strictly speaking unthinkable; to think the *multiple* impossibilities for thought designated by the term "AIDS"; to think the status of AIDS not only as object (in its objectness or objectity, its *Gegenstandlichkeit*), but also in and as the exigency that is its material objectivity; to think the impossibility of the object, but also the objectivity of its impossibility; to think AIDS as, and in, its material multiplicity, its material exigencies (both the multiplicity of its exigencies and the exigency of its multiplicity). In other words, I am trying to think the thought of AIDS as the *limit* that is at once the failure of thought and the sole condition of possibility for thought; I

do so because I am persuaded that any thinking or acting with respect to the AIDS pandemic that aspires to any effective *consequence*
must subject itself to such an onto-epistemological panic, not as a
putatively salutary propaedeutic humiliation (the discipline that
would subjectify us in disciplinary bondage), but as a *necessary* response to the exigency of the existential, the material force of the
Real of AIDS.

There is now a substantial body of work that testifies to, records,
and is itself part of the process by which the object we recognize
and sometimes claim to know as AIDS has been constituted, and is
continuously reconstituted, out of an amorphous terror.[5] This process, which has produced for the subject who is supposed to know
the massively overdetermined object called AIDS, is undoubtedly
necessary, and in any event unavoidable. But it has nevertheless not
been without its contradictions. For part of what has happened in
this constitution of an object for consciousness in and through material discursive practices, particularly in the past few years, has been
what might be termed the normalization, routinization, and, indeed, commodification of AIDS. AIDS has long since become big
business, not only for the pharmaceutical industry, for governmen-
tal regulatory and social service agencies, and for the health-care
industry, but also for those whose labor it is to produce knowledge,
for scientists, philosophers, historians, and sociologists among others. AIDS is now a career, the business of topical papers and books
produced by academics on the make, for example.

Concomitantly, the so-called phenomenon of AIDS has become very much part of the texture of the quotidian, central to our
commonsense perceptions of the way the world is, and thereby to
our sense of commonality. For example, many of our undergradu-
ate students have never known, and perhaps never will know, sex
without latex; we are now being urged to think of HIV seropositivity, and indeed of "AIDS itself," as a chronic condition on the
order of diabetes; we are, in short, becoming persuaded that AIDS
belongs to the normative rather than the extraordinary, that AIDS is
chronic rather than a crisis. We have erected, in place, perhaps, of
other erections, entire structures of intelligibility and comprehensi-

bility on and around the pandemic, structures that themselves render AIDS normative and routine: the business of AIDS, constructed and carried on around an impossible object, has become—like genocide, nuclear terror, racism, misogyny, and heteronormativity (or what I would prefer to call orthosexuality)—business as usual. The unthinkable has been rendered thinkable, the impossible possible, the extraordinary normative. And this process, however inevitable and in fact necessary it may be, is nevertheless at the same time a forgetting of the Real of AIDS, an avoidance of the exigencies with which the force of that Real confronts us, a refusal to think the limits of what can be thought, a disavowal of historicity. What is at stake here is a "something" rather more than epistemological bad faith, a "something" that is quite central to the constitution, validation, and valorization of our knowledges; that "something" might be called the aspiration to transcend the limit at which predication (and specifically every discourse on AIDS) exhausts itself in an infinite congestion of the proper, an aspiration to transcend the Real of AIDS, to transcend historicity—a transcendence that would be achieved through rendering AIDS comprehensible, and a grounding of that comprehensibility in ontology, in taking the objectness of AIDS to reside in the presumptive positivity of what is. In other words, neither a god nor the social sciences can save us now.[6] But perhaps salvation (transcendence) is beside the point; how, then—or rather, how *now*—might we begin to think the specific unthinkability, the determinate nontranscendent materiality, of AIDS?

In the first instance, I think we must work toward thinking of this impossible object that is called AIDS as a *multiplicity*. We must think the impossibility of the singular AIDS-object to be multiple, and that multiplicity to be central to both the objectness and objectivity of AIDS: the impossibility of the AIDS-object resides in its *originary* multiplicity. First, and perhaps most obviously, the phrase "Acquired Immune Deficiency Syndrome" refers precisely to a *syndrome*, which is to say, to a congeries of opportunistic (that is, *radically contingent*) infections: so-called "active" or "full-blown" AIDS is not a disease; there is no "AIDS virus." Indeed, scientific opinion

remains divided on whether the Human Immunodeficiency Virus is
singular; and there is mounting evidence that, even if it is a single
virus, "it" may be mutating. AIDS certainly, and HIV possibly,
are/is *multiple*. Second, and a large literature bears witness to the
fact, AIDS is not, and never has been, merely a medico-scientific
object; it has always already been at once also a social, political, economic, historical, philosophical, and literary object.[7] Which means
that AIDS was not, either logically or chronologically, *first of all* a
medico-scientific object that somehow *then* became an object for
other knowledges. This is perhaps obvious, but it bears emphasis
because it implies—necessarily I think—not merely that AIDS, *as
object and in its objectness*, is discursively constituted (a commonplace
in many quarters), but also that "it" does not exist in some primordial ontological viral plenitude, only subsequently subject to the
disciplines of knowing. Which means that *in* its multiplicity, and *as*
its multiplicity, it can bring down more than one house of epistemological cards: a jeux Descartes, indeed. Third, and equally obviously, perhaps, AIDS (so-called) is a very different object in Kin-
shasa than it is in New York, in Chang Mai than in San Francisco, in
Tokyo than in Port-au-Prince, for women than for men, and so
forth. But this "and so forth" is the *index*, not merely of a cultural
relativism, but also (and thereby) of the infinite proliferation of difference, the index of a limit where precisely because there is always,
with respect to the object, something *more* to be said, *nothing* has
been, or can definitively be said. This does not mean that we cannot, least of all that we should not, think and talk about AIDS; but
it does mean that such a thinking must *always also be something other*
than a subject thinking about an object. It is not that multiple interpretations coagulate around a singular object (in which case the
truth of AIDS would simply be—unaccountably—missing, as if the
AIDS-object were simply out of its ontological place), but that in its
radically originary multiplicity, AIDS gives the lie to every possible ontology, perhaps to the very possibility of ontology. There is
yet a further implication to this "cultural multiplicity" of the AIDS-
object: the urgent questions of racism, misogyny, heteronormativity,
"and so forth" can henceforth no longer be thought of as separate

"social problems," distinct from AIDS. For example, we live in a situation in which very few people indeed will identify themselves as racists. If such people themselves constituted the problem of racism, the problem (given a well-armed thought police) would soon be eradicated: we live, however, in a racist world without racists (in other words, racism is not *in the first instance* a psychological problem). My argument is that racism, misogyny, heteronormativity, "and so forth" are expressed nowhere but in structural determinations—for example, of AIDS policies. Conversely, and for purposes of the present argument more important, AIDS, by virtue of the originary multiplicity of the AIDS-object, cannot be considered apart from questions of racism, misogyny, heteronormativity, "and so forth."[8] This is not to say that they are somehow all the same thing; it is to say, however, that despite their quite heterogeneous genealogies, by virtue of their originary mutual imbrication, they structure and reinforce each *[an overlapping of -iles]* other: in this sense, the AIDS-object is not accidental.

If AIDS in its originary multiplicity thus disrupts the ontological as such, and if the term "AIDS" nevertheless marks one of the sites at which the Real in its existential materiality imposes an irrecusable exigency upon us, then it would seem necessary to specify this disruption *[not subject to objectivity]* as clearly as possible. I shall attempt to do so under four rubrics: the global (as something other than totality), the erotic (as zero-degree *aisthēsis*), historicity, and sociality. Which means, taken together, the political.

The Global

In order at least to begin to think AIDS in its globality, which would mean to think the global both as totality and as the simultaneous surpassing of every possible or ideal totality, as totalization and at the same time as the impossibility of totalization, therefore, we might consider the obvious.

First, there is nothing to suggest that either AIDS or the HIV seropositivity that is held to be the condition of possibility for the appearance of AIDS is a unique phenomenon. Nothing suggests that there exist no other viruses, perhaps considerably less fragile and even more readily transmitted but equally deadly, that are capable of achieving pandemic status: whether or not AIDS is the first pandemic of its kind, there is no reason to believe that it will be the last. Which means that, even were we to entertain fantasies of a heroic science discovering the magic bullet (the lost object of desire if ever there was one), the specific impossibilities with which AIDS confronts us would yet appear with a perhaps even greater virulence. One might as well suppose that nuclear terror disappeared with Fat Man and Little Boy. In other words, we are confronted with radically different material conditions of possibility for existence.

Second, AIDS is obviously global in that it ("it" in its multiple singularity and singular multiplicity) is truly *pandemic*; there is quite literally nowhere on the globe that is "outside" the pandemic. This is undoubtedly an effect of the radically and irreversibly changed material conditions of possibility for viral transmission brought about by the urban explosion, the incessant movement of people and peoples, the virtual simultaneity of such movement among urban centers across the great air bridges that connect them in an infinite hyphenation, and so forth. Technology has made the Human Immunodeficiency Virus the world's first true cosmopolitan. Very schematically, we might therefore say that AIDS and its allotropes are global both synchronically and diachronically, and are so precisely in the very movement that renders the mutually exclusive opposition of synchrony and diachrony unstable.[9] From these rather obvious observations we must, I think, pursue certain irrecusable possibilities.

Globality, I have said, indicates both totality *and* the excess, surplus, or surpassing of every possible totality, both a necessary totalization and an equally necessary impossibility of totalization. We cannot have done with the category of totality or the movement of totalization (a concept, a movement absolutely necessary to the thought of the very possibility of the social and human sciences) precisely because the AIDS pandemic totalizes in an integrated viral relationality, at least possibly, otherwise heterogeneous (or even het-

eronomous) "elements."〉AIDS unites such "elements" in the totality of an annihilation-in-common, in a technological mass death,
in utter nihility. In effect, AIDS is a holocaust; in that this holocaust bespeaks totality-as-utter-nihility, it belongs to the order of
other holocausts, actualized or merely promised, such as nuclear terror, ecological disaster, and previous (or concurrent) genocides. I
do not think there is any possibility for a consequent thinking with
regard to the AIDS pandemic without this thought of totalization,
any more than there is with regard to nuclear terror, ecological disaster, or other genocides.〈But in each case, such a totality must be
thought of as a totality present only in its material effects. In other
words, there is a totalization at work here, but because the totality as
such is only present in its effects, it is by that token absent for consciousness and knowing; the "global" here, then, marks the thought
of a material effectivity.〉

　　Globality, however, also denominates the excess, surplus, or surpassing of any totality that could be posited as the privileged object, albeit in a certain ideality, of and for consciousness and knowing. AIDS is global, I have said, in that it is pandemic; there is no
"outside" of AIDS, "it" is a phenomenon of mass death (which is
not a death-in-general: no one has ever died "in general"). Now
the fact that there is no "outside" of AIDS, the globality of AIDS,
does not necessarily mean that everyone will eventually succumb
to AIDS-related causes. But it does necessarily imply that AIDS de-
fies the logic of separation and containment. Here, "globality" signifies nothing but a certain *material* impossibility of separation and
containment. The Human Immunodeficiency Virus is the first true
cosmopolitan, respecting neither geographic, cultural, sexual, class,
nor racial boundaries; the only boundaries the virus respects are
those of the skin, bleach, latex, and nonoxynol-9. Yet the institutional, political, economic, and cultural histories of the pandemic
are histories of truly abject failures to contain AIDS effectively
within what are often enough taken to be virtually natural, indeed
ontological, and above all *practical* separations. And this both in terms
of its etiology and its epidemiology. At both levels (and it is precisely here that the distinction between public and private is re-

vealed to be essentially stupid), AIDS discourse has by and large sustained a fatal nostalgia for the clean and proper body, which is also a no less fatal nostalgia for the clean and proper body politic.

⟨At the level of the individual body, which is thus exposed in its erotic relations to be primordially political, it has taken the form of a thoroughly moralist discourse on safer sex, a discourse that reveals its essential moralism in the concept of the so-called "innocent victim."⟩ (I must hurry parenthetically to say here, and first of all, that I am not advocating the abandonment of safer-sex education or practices; neither, however, am I advocating their necessary imposition.) Of all that could be said here, of all that must be said here, I would merely say that this moralism, which extends far beyond a certain puritanism, assumes the pleasures of the body to be unessential, immoderate, excessive, and therefore deniable; it assumes pleasure to be negotiable within an autarkic economy of prophylaxis. Ultimately, it assumes the mere instrumentality of the body, which in its mere instrumentality subsists in its separation from all other bodies, rather than as a site of the primordial imbrication with others and *as* otherness. What is being rejected here is the primordially *erotic* historico-socio-*politicality* of the body. Above all, there is mounting evidence that this moralist discourse on the clean and proper body simply is not working, either because condoms, dental dams, and clean works for IV drug users are not available, or out of what is called "choice."[10]

The logics of separation and containment also operate at the epidemiological level (the etiological and epidemiological levels are, of course, from the first mutually imbricated). This is most obvious in the institutional politics of the nation-state, in the nostalgia for a clean and proper body politic, in notions of cultural immunity (where cultural community supposedly provides a preemptive cultural immunity), and this whether culture is taken to be constituted by race, ethnicity, gender, class, or sexuality. There have been and, of course, continue to be attempts to sustain the separations of such cultural immunities through a series of institutional practices that function as a kind of cultural inoculation. I am thinking (for example: the list is by no means exhaustive) of U.S. immigration policies (particularly with regard to Haiti), of enforced quarantine of HIV positives (as proposed in the United States and apparently enforced in Cuba), of the refusal of New York State to countenance a needle-exchange program, of proposals for the tattooing, sterilization, and castration of HIV positives, of prison policies, of calls for mandatory testing, and of a blind refusal even to acknowledge that the problem exists. It is in these policies and practices, *as well as in the logics of separation and containment that sustain such policies and practices*, that the AIDS pandemic is in effect genocidal. For what these practices and logics openly acknowledge is that the (entirely fantasmatic) clean and proper body politic is maintained only in the processes of the exclusion of an expendable social surplus comprised of people and peoples of color, sex workers, IV drug users, and queers; the exclusion, that is to say, of all those of us whose bodies are encoded as excessively and preternaturally erotic, all those of us who are said to be excessively devoted to the practices of pleasure; all those of us who are held to be therefore incapable of distinguishing with any eroto-epistemological surety between self and other. Our very corporeality is taken to be at once the locus of immoderate pleasures and therefore that of contagion, impurity, and death. In these practices and logics, we have at once the closely allied structures of fascination and disavowal—a classic fascism, to be sure. What I want to emphasize here is that this is not merely a psychological phenomenon. This amounts to a certain fear of the failure of separation, a fear of noncontainment, a fear of the global, a fear of difference (which means a fear of history and the social).

I must emphasize that the logics of separation and containment are the refusal of any possible logic of difference. The logics of separation and containment are fundamentally logics of identity, logics of the antithesis of particular and universal, logics that exclude you on the basis of who you putatively are, or even logics of *what* you do (rather than a logic of *how* you do what you do, a logic of use and need, of *Brauch*). The logics of containment and separation acknowledge a separation founded in identity only as particularity, as particular instances of universality, never calling into question the universality of the category of "identity." One is separate on the basis of one's identity, but, because the category of identity is never interrogated, the putative fact that one *has* and/or *is* an identity is never questioned; identity is therefore what one has in common with everyone else—a relation of sameness. The categories of particularity and universality are complicit precisely *because* they are antithetical and therefore hold out the promise of integration within the totality (I pursue this below in Chapter 2). Hegelian-to-be-sure: more-important, they are central to liberal humanism's logic of integration, the acknowledgment of difference only if it be recuperated in the Same. It is a logic of totality as the integration of apparently different phenomena on the basis of their essential similitude. The global, however, is the radical impossibility of totalization because it is an attempt to think the *thought of* a singularity irreducible to concepts of identity, individuality, or "subjectivity," and therefore of a singularity that can never be recuperated in the unity of an integrated totality. The singular can never be the object for any knowledge. Neither particular nor element, the singular necessarily always figures as the excess or surplus of totality, as that which is rejected or excluded in order to achieve the integration of the totality. The global, therefore, is a contradiction, at once a necessary totalization (insofar as the totality is always present in its effects) and the impossibility of totality (insofar as it indicates the nonrelation, the difference, of infinite singularity). We are required to think the global as a contradiction, in its unthinkability. For what we call thought (although not necessarily for thinking), this is impossible; but this impossibility is a limit, the *thought of* what cannot be thought. Not even the dialectic can save us now.

The Erotic

I want to attempt to specify what I have put very generally and formally here. Indissociable from this globality, it seems to me, are three terms that articulate the global character of what is called AIDS, and that I hope will clarify the point I am trying to make. Each term is central to any consideration of AIDS, yet each designates a concrete impossibility for knowing, which is to say that none can be taken to be an *object for* knowledge. I want briefly to attend to questions of the erotic, of historicity, and of sociality as disruptions of any possibility for onto-epistemological certitude, in order to say that the impossibility of the AIDS-object in its objectivity calls into radical question the very possibility of the idea of the social and human sciences, in order to suggest that there is still plenty to do for those of us who used to be called social scientists; that that something to do will *not* keep us off the streets; and that that "something to do," if we abandon the narcoleptic comforts of our epistemophiliac business as usual, might be a political "intervention."

Undoubtedly, we have all observed how a certain disgusted fascination has located the origin (not only beginning but essence) of AIDS in what is taken to be the preternaturally erotic, in the material bodies of people and peoples of color, the sex worker, the queer, the IV drug user. We are all too familiar with an epidemiological construction of the pandemic that situates its origin (and therefore its essential immutable nature) in sub-Saharan Africa, and its development (which is to say its noncontainment) in Haiti and the brothels of Southeast Asia; the introduction of HIV to the clean and proper (i.e., white) bodies politic of the United States and Europe is attributed to the IV drug user and the (essentially promiscuous) gay male. It has not gone unnoticed that this construction of the pandemic repeats what are by now very tired, but nonetheless virulently racist, constructions of Africa, the Caribbean, and Southeast Asia as realms of unbridled, barely contained, eroticism and pestilence, against which only the heroic vigilance of our contemporary Schweitzers at the NIH and CDC can provide prophylaxis. Here, the fatality of the pandemic is held to reside in erotic congress with the natural other, in the failure of cultural containment.

Concomitantly, and this concomitance is rigorously allotropic, etiological constructions of AIDS situate the origins of HIV infection, and therefore the essential fatality of the body, in material erotic relations: in IV drug use and in the incorporation of polluted alien blood, semen, vaginal fluids, and breast milk (the status of sweat, saliva, and tears is still being contested). An entire semiology has been constructed here: the fatally erotic relation is construed in terms of taking what belongs least of all to the property and propriety of one's own body into the innermost recesses of the privacy of the clean and proper body. (The incorporation of the radically other becomes the very mortality of the proper identity of the self; the other *is* my finitude. It is the transgression of a proper identity (what Freud would have called the ego) that not only brings but incarnates death. The price of disrupting the opposition of outside to inside is death. Further, these transgressions occur at particular sites, the body's lamellae—the puncture wounds of the needle, the mouth, the vagina, the tip of the penis, and above all, the anus. (In all cases we are dealing with surfaces that are both inside and outside, and therefore neither "inside" nor "outside," sites at which the putative corporeal integrity of the so-called self is always already ambiguous, sites that are always already wounds and therefore susceptible to infection by the other; indeed, by otherness "itself." Finally, this erotic congress with others is a matter, *the* matter in its materiality, of flows, of fluids and fluidity, of the radical instability (by which I mean an instability that is always also something other than an accident that befalls stability) of flux. All of this is what is said must be prevented, both epidemiologically and etiologically, in order to confront the AIDS pandemic.

Now in this conception, whether it be of the clean and proper (i.e., HIV negative) bodies or of clean and proper bodies politic, prophylaxis—not only against HIV infection, but against death itself—is conceived in terms of containment, of course, but it does so by regarding the body as *nothing but* its instrumentality. In other words, as long as the erotic is conceived to be a simple transaction or negotiation between an unproblematic self and a disgusting but nonetheless essentially unproblematic other, between ontologically primordial identities, then HIV transmission can only be conceived of in terms of the instrumentality of the body, subject therefore to engineering, to various regimes of truth. But this is to attempt in a certain prophylaxis to occlude the erotic altogether, which is in the same occlusion to attempt a prophylaxis against historicity and sociality.

This is also to relegate the erotic to the place of a regrettably *recidivism - habitual relapse into crime* (as)

unhygienic "natural" necessity in a relatively crude functionalism, at best to the status of a recidivist call of the wild, against which we have unhappily not been entirely successful in stopping our ears, those other lamellae. And this despite various explicit protestations to the contrary from the less thoughtful advocates of safer sex. I want to suggest that a consideration of the erotic, in the *dimensions* I have just sketched so hastily, is absolutely central to any *consequent* consideration of the AIDS pandemic. I am not going to offer an alternative definition of the erotic, as if the erotic could be securely, that is, universally, differentiated from the nonerotic; I do not want to ask what the erotic *is*, a necessarily impossible question. (Parenthetically, I should remark that what is at issue here is not the question of "personal taste," which would assume the regularity of a relation between aisthēsis and the aesthetic, between sensuousness and representation, *and* would also assume that the erotic ultimately belongs to the putative coherence of what is called "experience.") Rather, I want to ask what is at stake when it is the erotic that is at stake? What is at stake *in* the erotic being at stake? In a word: everything.)

First and last, what is at stake is materiality, the material relation of what cannot yet be objectified but that has always already been objectified as bodies, to what can never yet be objectified but that has always already been objectified as the world. Materiality designates here what might be called a "zero-degree aisthēsis," the sensuousness of an unobjectifiable Real in its prior or originary objectivity, a material aisthēsis that is radically always also something other than the object of and for perception, predication, and judgment. Materiality designates a relation insofar as our only possibility for positing the existence of a material Real resides in a passage through affective apprehension, perception, objectification, predication, and judgment (through an aesthetics, therefore) but "materiality" also designates a nonrelation insofar as the existence of the Real does not depend upon the apprehension thereof and is therefore always also something other than its objectness, a nonrelation insofar as zero-degree aisthēsis necessarily figures as the surplus or excess of every possible aesthetics, and thus of aesthetics as such.

Materiality therefore designates a nonrelating relation, an impossibility or limit for any thought grounded in the logics of non-contradiction.

Now this nonrelating relation designated by the term "materiality" can only be situated in fact in a present, a Now. It is possible only to imagine or conceive of a materiality situated in what is called the past or what is called the future; but the materiality of past or future is only a materiality situated in the past's present or the future's present—situated, that is to say, in ideality. Further, materiality, a nonrelating relation situated in the radical immediacy of a Now, in the very presence of the present, necessarily and thereby designates a disjunct simultaneity, an impossibility of totalization, and this because the Now, the presence of the present, the force that *is* the Real, is radically ungraspable for thought. The erotic in its essential materiality (an oxymoronic formulation, to be sure) is, in the fulguration of the Now, simultaneously absolute presence and absolute absence, and also the absence of presence, the presence of that absence. I am never more present to myself than in erotic relation, nor more other to myself than in the nonrelationality of the erotic. In other words, the erotic in its materiality can only transpire in what philosophy calls the *ekstases* of temporality, in the nothing-but-nowness of the Now—in the ecstasies of music, dancing, *play*, and in what is called sex—in the "free time" that is the very motility or movement, the very transitivity, of be-ing, in the time that is *at once* the impossible ground of the possibility of time *and* the surplus or excess of every constituted temporality.[11]

Among the many implications here, two are of particular importance for the present argument. First, this means that materiality and the erotic are essentially immemorial, a parenthetical syncope in the very possibility of narrative linearity, knowing neither "past" nor "future" in their essential ideality. And it is precisely in the syncopation of here-and-nowness, the immemorial presentness, of the nonrelating relation of the erotic in its materiality, that the etiological and epidemiological origin, and hence essence, of AIDS is lost, an erotic materiality we are summoned, in the interest of the clean and proper body politic, to deny. Which is why it will always be impossible to write the history of AIDS.[12] Secondly, and concomitantly, the erotic in its materiality is also without teleology. The play of erotic materiality is without purpose, and refers beyond itself to nothing save the infinite play of what is; which also means that the erotic is without instrumentality. Now this absence of telos, an absence that is not a deprivation, constitutes the erotic nonrelation as what Freud termed perversity.

Here I must again emphasize that the immemorial perversity of the erotic in its materiality necessarily, for consciousness and for thought, always figures as a surplus or excess. Which means not only that there is no outside of erotic materiality, that our erotic nonrelating relation in the materiality of what is is not optional, but also that the erotic is not an alternative, a kind of *jouissance* wherein self becomes orgasm and world itself an amniotic flux. Rather, the immemorial perversity of the erotic, situated in the ekstases of temporality, necessarily figures as both the condition of possibility for and as the limit of any phenomenological apprehension whatsoever, including the phenomenological apprehension of self in autoaffectivity; in short, the erotic is not what is called an experience, which happens to a perceiving, knowing subject. Thus, there can be no phenomenology of the erotic, the erotic is the aporia of subjectivity. Because the erotic is a limit, an aporia, it cannot be known in itself; the aporia of the erotic can only ever be approached as the failure of phenomenological apprehension, phenomenology is the necessary passage to its own, indeed its "ownmost," impossibility. But at this limit, a limit we can only approach through a phenomenology, however informal, but a limit at which we always already are, is also the place (a kind of ontological lamella) where the distinction between self and other is rendered essentially and originarily unstable (an instability that is not the degeneration of a prior stability). It is a "moment" of absolute communion and communication, but also of the absolute failure of communion and communication, a "moment" simultaneously of ultimate integration with and of ultimate separation from the other. In the ultimate becoming-other of the "little death," one nevertheless dies alone. And this necessarily implies, of course, that the erotic, in its existential materiality, confounds the subject/object distinction. The obscurity of all this is clear enough. What is important here seems to me to follow unavoidably: that the erotic, our existential implication in the materiality of what is, is without relation to truth. Or rather, the relation of the erotic to truth *is* its nonrelation to truth; better yet, the truth of the erotic is its being outside and beyond truth.

Historicity

These, then, are among the questions at stake when it is the erotic that is at stake, the questions at stake when it is the origin and essence of AIDS that are at stake, when it is therefore the truth of AIDS that is at stake. As with the origin of AIDS, so too with its telos. If the origin of AIDS is situated in the immemorial perversity of the erotic, the telos of AIDS, a telos that by the terms of a well-known logic is always already incarnate in the essentiality of the generative origin, resides in the degeneration and dissolution of death, in utter abjection. When it is a matter of AIDS, when it is *the* matter of AIDS, as the force of the Real in its very existentiality, origin, essence, and truth can only be thought as certain resistances to thought, a thought figured as the erotic, a thought that can be thought only *as* and *through* the failure of consciousness, perception, and thought. So, too, can the absolute destitution and abject finitude that is death—in other words, the radical historicity that can only be grounded in the materiality of what is—only be thought, when it is a question of the historical, as the ultimate failure of historicization. The thought of historicity is the acknowledgment of the ultimate incapacity of historical consciousness to account for, or give meaning to, the utter destitution, the traumatic sensuous senselessness of what is in its materiality. The thought of historicity, as both the condition of possibility for, and aporetic limit of, historical consciousness, the exteriority or alterity that is at the heart of historical consciousness, can only be thought as a surplus or excess produced at the limit—the Real—where prediction exhausts itself in the infinite congestion of singularity (as in the recitation of names on the

[handwritten marginalia: prolepsis: the representation of something in the future as if it already existed. : anticipation]

anniversary of Kristalnacht or at exhibitions of the AIDS quilt, for example), in the necessary incompletion of the work of mourning and historicization, that is to say.[13]

The dissolution, disintegration, or degradation unto death figured for us as AIDS cannot be narrated according to the teleology of fate or destiny (as the wages of the erotic, for example) precisely because AIDS in its singular multiplicity figures as a random series of opportunistic—which is to say, *contingent*—infections. Again, the thought of this radical contingency leads us inexorably to the impossibility of a historical phenomenological apprehension, the impossibility of the determination of a tragic narrativity in and by a teleology. Recall that the work of mourning, including the proleptic work of mourning that produces the so-called "AIDS victim," is a process by which the dead are rendered radically other, a process simultaneously of dissociation and objectification whereby a certain "that" is recognized to be nothing more than an abject object—dead meat. At once a labor of abjectification and objectification, the work of mourning historicizes the dead, giving "historical" meaning to death, and in historicizing the dead, occludes the traumatic insistence of the Real, the radical nontranscendence that is historicity. And this occlusion, this historicization, this work of mourning, putatively constitutes a redemption. Moreover, what is at work in the work of mourning is the Imaginary constitution of identity *in* and *as Bildung*. Every historicization holds out the promise of intelligibility and sense, but it is precisely in this promise of intelligibility and sense, in issuing a promissory note to be drawn on the account of an ideal transcendental subjectivity (and what is transcended here is the historicity of a materiality that is every intelligibility's condition of possibility), that historicization becomes Bildung. In other words, we are talking about the rhetorical constitution of community: you and I, as it were, we have access to a rationality that would render radical contingency intelligible; in that shared access, you and I become a "we." In this work of historicization, at once *Arbeit, oeuvre*, and *Bildung*, the unspeakable is spoken, the unimaginable imagined, the unthinkable thought, the unrepresentable represented—and the unbearable rendered bearable for an "us" constituted in what is presumptively the communion of communication.

And yet an entire literature, which is not the so-called "AIDS literature," testifies to the impossibility of a successful accomplishment of the work of mourning, the work of historicization. I think, for example, of the work of David Wojnarowicz or of Marlon Riggs; the refusal of the status of the victim by People Living With AIDS in the Denver Principles of 1983; the recitation of names at displays of the AIDS quilt; the institution, associated with ACT UP, of the political funeral.[14] In each case, it seems to me, we are recalled to an attention to the utter destitution of Spirit, the radical impossibility of transcendence, the absolute historicity, of what is: not even the historian can save us now. Now this insistence upon the necessary incompletion of the work of mourning, this refusal of historicization and the redemption in "historical" meaning that it offers, this rejection of the very possibility of even an ideal transcendental subjectivity, can only be undertaken *through* the work of mourning, the passages of historicization, the desire that informs the aspiration to transcendental subjectivity. We cannot think destitution of Spirit or the radical historicity of what is in the force of their immediacy, in the presence and presentness of their nontranscendental materiality. These terms—historicity, materiality, destitution, nontranscendence—can only be thought as the *traces* of what it is impossible to think. As the proper name (indeed, as language itself), the trace marks the place of an absence. The trace is not a representation of a presence, but the indication of the impossibility of representing the Real: the trace is the index of the radical insufficiency of the word. The trace, and the word as trace, is what haunts language, inevitably bespeaking an absence; insofar as it bespeaks a *certain* absence, it is the presence of that absence, the presence of that absent presence (not relation, but the relation of nonrelation): in short, the trace is a ghost, the very figure of ideality, and thereby of Spirit. Spirit (*Geist*)—which is to say, ideality as condition of possibility for any thinking whatsoever—is the ghost (*Geist*) that haunts all thought, the memorial of the Real.[15]

The Social

The trace, therefore, is not a communication, but rather marks an essential syncope in the very possibility *for* communication, and gives the lie to any thought of community as established in the communion of communication, in the intersubjective recognition of similitude. The trace marks the impossibility of establishing an ontologically grounded shared epistemology, a shared historiographical understanding of the Real (for example). It is for this reason that the refusal of the work of mourning and historicization in a number of practices, the refusal of meaning and intelligibility, the refusal of every soteriology, is also a refusal of community as constituted in the reproduction of the Same, in the shared understanding of sympathy and empathy. The refusal of the historicizing work of mourning is at the same time the refusal of the redemptive consolations of every humanism. These refusals give the lie to the logic of integration that is the ideological ground of humanism and, indeed, humanitarianism. For humanism projects an Imaginary totality—the human community—within which the essentially erotic abject is reintegrated *only on condition that that abjection is accepted or in fact affirmed.* One is accepted into the community of the "we" only insofar as one accepts one's essentially passive objectness (as the abject object of a proleptic work of mourning), only insofar as one rejects one's difference, one's singular otherness. Which is no integration at all, of course. Thus, as I have already noted, a certain social surplus—the IV drug user, the person of color, the sex worker, the queer—is produced in order to maintain humanism's "society," constituted in the genetic, viral, and bacteriological law and order of the clean and proper body, as *the* privileged community of the Same. And, as I have also emphasized under the rubric of the global, this so-called social surplus is not merely the index of the proliferation of objects before the panoptic Gaze of a magisterial transcendental subjectivity (the social scientist-engineer); much more radically, it is the endless proliferation, in destitution, of difference itself, signifying the radical impossibility of constituting "society" as totality.

If the objectification of the social constructs a putative totality called "society" and the historicization of the Real consists of a donation of meaning, taken together they are unavoidably and originarily a transcendental *forgetting* of the erotic, destitute, materiality of the Real in its historicity; if representation necessarily occludes *what* is presumptively being represented; if humanism constitutes the human community only in enacting and *enforcing* certain exclusions under the banner of integration; then must the erotic in its immemorial perversity, historicity in its radical destitution, the Real in its resistance to representability, the AIDS-object in its ultimately unobjectifiable multiplicity, all bespeak what would be first and last an existential *entropy*, an ultimate degeneration, the radical failure of any possibility for community? In a word: yes. And this anarchic entropy is unavoidable.

The Political

There are four themes that need to be broached here in order to argue that this thought is not a conclusion, an absolutely passive nihilism that would ultimately leave everything unchanged. On the contrary, this thought of an absolute indifference is the sole possibility for thinking the thought of difference. If we cannot think the thought of the erotic, of materiality, of historicity, of sociality as this entropic proliferation of infinite difference, then we cannot think of *any* difference in its singularity. Without the thought of historicity, it is impossible to think what might be historical: one cannot think of the radical difference between a past and present without a thought of the trace as the mark of the absence of presence that is our historicity; one cannot think of the radical difference between a present and a futurity without the thought of historicity. To be blunt: every revolution is in its essence a nihilism. Or, another slogan: politicality, as the desire for an encounter with otherness, and therefore the possibility of any politics whatsoever, is in its essence *erotic*. It is this that what is called AIDS gives us to think: without the thought of the "historical space" of an entropic nihility, the thought of an essential motility, of the limit-situation (and of "situation" *as* limit), of the despairing destitution of existential singularity, then it is impossible to think the very possibility of the ethico-political. We must recognize that the ethical can only be grounded in the impossibility of grounding an ethics in ontology. In other words: being is the very unjustifiability of being, being is violence, the Law is always in its instauration of necessity illegal. Any ethics that would be something other than an adjudication must think its own condition of possibility to be outside the Law. It is precisely to such an ethicality that certain actions of ACT UP might summon us; conversely, such an outlaw ethicality summons us to act up.[16]

Second, a thinking the thought of the erotic, of materiality, of historicity, of sociality (or the global) can never reduce the erotic, materiality, historicity, or sociality—in short, the global—to concepts. This thinking of all that is involved in thinking the thought of AIDS is not to think a concept, that which as a propaedeutic gesture might be reduced to the status of an axiom in a theoretical *askēsis*, thus both validating and valorizing the production of a knowledge adequate, precisely, to its concept. Such indeed would be a project that would betray its animating impulse, for it would establish the concept as the outside of historicity, as the sign of a transcendental subjectivity that miraculously survives the depredations of historicity. And this means that we can never have done with thinking the thought of historicity: thinking the thought can never produce the concept. This is to say, this is a thinking that is in search neither of an object, although it is not without its objects, nor of a method, although it is not without its procedures. And this is, precisely, a historical relation to what is presumptively the thought that is being thought. There is a major implication here: such a thinking, which is to think *within* the radical instability of the impossibility of thought, is to refuse to "play the game" of the struggle for hegemonic authority or the hermeneutic "conflict of interpretations." It never amounts to a decision between contesting explanations of the world, or the methodologies that supposedly constitute the persuasiveness of any such explanation or interpretation. To put it otherwise, such a thinking constitutes a refusal to posit a utopia, an alternative totality: the categorical imperative is inoperative here. Indeed, one might well think here of an erotics of thinking. Now, while such a thinking is without a telos, it is not without its effects, because it is first of all an *intervention* in a "situation" (which is always a limit, the limit imposed by our historicity). First of all, there is no chance that somehow, suddenly, miraculously, everyone is going to attend to the possibilities of this thinking: it is necessarily a guerrilla action, which attempts in the first instance, and essentially, to open a *space for* politicality and critique, a space that is increasingly being foreclosed, and nowhere more so than in AIDS discourse. Second, such interventions are the *relation* of a thinking that refuses to be a thought in search of the disciplinary authorizations provided by method, object, or concept *to* the force of an "outside," the force of certain determinate exigencies (such as what is called AIDS), which thereby designate the force of exigency "itself." If intervention designates that relation, that nonrelating relation, then the ethico-political register of such a thinking is not that of a post-festum implication or effect. What would be in question, rather, is a certain effectivity, immanent in the rigorous transgressiveness of thinking as nomadic, guerrilla intervention. Thinking acts up by raising hell.

The third congeries of themes opened up by the practice of this thinking with regard to AIDS revolves around what might be called the status of representation. If it is a question of the Real, then it would take little reflection—or perhaps, on the contrary, it would require infinite reflection—to realize that the status of representation is no longer, if ever it was, merely that of a mimesis to be judged according to the accuracy of its correspondence to what is called reality, and thereby its purchase upon the truth. For we must realize that the distinction between the Real and the Imaginary is not a distinction between the true and the false; one and the same image can belong simultaneously to the Real and to the Imaginary. In representation, an object—AIDS, for instance—can be both the trace of a Real that resists comprehensibility absolutely *and* the occlusion of that radical incomprehensibility in its status as an Imaginary object (the object, that is to say, with which one identifies, or—in disgust, fascination, and disavowal—refuses to identify, thus identifying with and as that refusal). But it is of the first importance to note that in the case of the AIDS-object, it is in no case a matter of substituting a truer, more "realistic" object or image, but of acknowledging the disruptions of the structures of the representations of which such an object is the occasion. In the case of the AIDS-object, *by virtue of its status in the Real*, it is not a matter of identification, as either the "that's me" of specular jubilation or the "I am not that" of an essentially paranoid disavowal. Also in question, therefore, are the identificatory structures of the Imaginary as they pertain to what is called education. It is very widely assumed, albeit sometimes with very great sophistication, that education, not excepting "AIDS education," through identification with the Imaginary object (the "human community," for example, or more generally a subject that comes to subjectivity in supposedly recognizing itself in its representations), produces a good, critical citizenry, a citizenry that, on the basis of authorized knowledges, feels the right feelings, thinks the right thoughts, and thereby cannot but feel good about itself. To emphasize the obvious: we do not discover our clean and proper body (politic) about which we feel so good and *then* subject it to representation; rather, in education, we identify ourselves with a certain clean and proper body presented *as if* in its integral specularity, a mythic identification that occludes the fact of our utter lack of specularity. In the time of AIDS, we are all of us vampires. Not even education can save us now.[17]

The fourth and final thematics that, as absolute exigency, is given to us to think when it is AIDS we are attempting to think, concerns the questions of community. We know, if not well enough, at least too well, the horrors a conception of community constituted in the recognition of an intersubjective similitude is apparently willing to countenance in the name of and as humanism. We also know, although perhaps less well, that this insistence upon our commonality is not without its necessity, for such is the toll exacted for our every attempt to speak to one another: language demands of us a forgetting, however grudging, of differences and of difference. It is nevertheless entirely unclear why the minimal communication we might persuade ourselves we accomplish in the communion said to constitute community should require the global holocausts of an epoch we too easily claim as our own. Why the invocation of what was once called the "brotherhood of man" should require innumerable genocides for its realization, why human community would require the hecatomb *for* and *as* its consummation are questions that belong essentially to the obscurities of what we too easily invoke as our histories, histories of the essential bankruptcy, the essential fraudulence, of humanism.

And yet, and yet: there remains—perhaps—a desire for an encounter with otherness, which in a dangerously generous gesture might be conceived to have been the animating impulse, the compassion, belonging to that of which humanism has been such a sorry expression. That compassion bespeaks a being-in-common grounded in the absolute groundlessness of the utter destitution of an entropic anarchy, a being-in-common of the abject damned, a community constituted in difference rather than grounded in the Same. But we have hardly begun to think with regard to a community constituted in, and indeed as, difference. Can community be constituted in the *failure* of communication, which is to say, with the death of the singular other in view? Might it not be the incessant syncopations in communication, syncopations that always displace us from the locus of the Law (thus displacing us, unprepared, in the atopic vulnerability of love), that constitute our only communion? Might it not be a *certain* impossibility of understanding that opens us to the very otherness of difference? But for essential and essentially historical reasons, we have hardly begun to think the thought of such a being-in-common. Yet such a being-in-common, such a compassion (which would be neither sympathy, empathy, nor pity), is the insistence of an irrecusable *demand* in the time of AIDS. With every suspicion of the rhetoric of interpellation, it must be said that this constitutes a *call* (which is at the same time a scream of abject terror), a call that summons us from beyond every possible horizon to what I can only term, for there is as yet no word adequate to indicate what must be thought here, the "ethical." Of what that ethicality might consist belongs, however, to whatever futurity may yet remain to us.

CHAPTER 2

First Excursus on the Divine Right of the Historian

> Not all relations to history can be scientifically objectified and given a place in science, and it is precisely the essential ones that cannot. Historical science can never establish the historical relation to history.
>
> —Martin Heidegger, *An Introduction to Metaphysics*

It is in and by the very act of what is called the "scholarly communication" of what we are doing that we historians constitute ourselves, for ourselves, as a scholarly community. It is not what we say we do, but the saying of what we say we do, that brings us together. Of course, we all know, and tend to insist rather strenuously upon the fact, that whatever community we may achieve is in no wise a community constituted according to a consensus regarding one or another specific historical interpretation. But we historians—by which I mean not only those of us who presumptively enjoy a professional franchise, but also all those who seek, both inside and outside the academy, a certain authorization in the very invocation of "the historical" or, indeed, of "History itself"—we do rather tend to assume a certain consensus, that a certain community exists with respect to the ontological, epistemological (what I shall refer to as the onto-epistemological) conditions of possibility for historiographical inquiry, representation, and interpretation. By and large, we tend to assume that an invocation of "History itself" is the sufficient and unproblematic ground of our historiographical epistemophilia. It is precisely in taking our own conditions of possibility for granted, in assuming that "there is" something called history that might be the object for our investigations, in the frequently voiceless but nevertheless audible invocation of "History itself," that we in fact imagine our community to have always already been instituted. In taking our onto-epistemological conditions of possibility for granted, we take our existence as community for granted. We assume, that is to say, that we know what we are talking about when we use this term "history." (Again, I remind you that I am talking in the first instance about a generalized invocation of history that includes but is not limited to professional historiography. That there are exceptions to this generalization might almost go without saying.) At this level—at the level of an assumed congruence of the ontological and the epistemological, a congruence that grounds consensual community—historical investigation, representation, and interpretation are *not* in crisis. But it is precisely to the extent that we avoid the possibility of crisis, the critical possibility that *is* onto-epistemological crisis, and thereby a crisis in the institution of communities, that we forfeit the possibility of making what we do a practice.

Insofar as it is a question that is central to the argument of the present project, I shall return repeatedly to this extremely problematic question of the rhetorical constitution or institution of community. But in order to be able to return to this question, it is first of all necessary to say what it is I think I am doing, in spite of, or perhaps because of, the fact that it is finally impossible to know, in any strong sense of the term, what one is in fact doing.

What I want, as a "historian," to be doing, what I think I am doing, is concerned with the question of practice. And the question of practice is a question I have never yet, and perhaps shall always have never yet, been able to pose in a form adequate to what it asks; perhaps, indeed, the question of practice is singularly the question we shall never know how to ask. For to suggest that we might adequately pose the question would suggest that the world, as totality, is, at least ideally, fully intelligible; thus, there can be no general theory of practice. Nevertheless, and contradictorily, the question of practice is also that question to which one has always already perforce responded, precisely because practice can never wait for its adequate theory. And perhaps this contradiction—that one is always already summoned to answer a question that one can never adequately formulate—is somehow essential to questions of practice and praxis. But one is undoubtedly in any case obliged to make a first approach to the question of practice in as straightforward a manner as possible. Here, then, is a statement of what I am doing, what I want to be doing, when it is a question of practice: I want to *think* (which is not to *know*) what a historical, political practice—as a nontranscendent, nonneutral intervention in a singular situation—or in that singularity that *is* a "situation"—might be. More specifically, I want to think what a historical, political practice interested in, or oriented toward, a future that would be something other than a continuity with, or maintenance of, the present, might be. For me, each term in this formulation is, perhaps necessarily, obscure. What I would like to do in what follows is to attempt to give some rigor to that obscurity, to understand why that obscurity may in fact be necessary and essential. If we can never finally know what we are doing, perhaps we can nonetheless attempt to know why we do not know what we are doing.

I pursue this question of practice in this excursus by means of what I hope is a politically attentive reading of certain texts; I do so in an attempt to achieve the rigor imposed by attention to the specificity of certain formulations, certain textual and rhetorical strategies, certain practices. I want thereby to avoid the hermeneutic strategy of attempting to recuperate an essential intention or meaning that would putatively lie beyond the texts, an intention or meaning that would putatively be immanent in the texts. In addition to general theoretical considerations, which have everything to do with the historicity of thought, there are in the present instance specific historical considerations that effectively block any strategy of hermeneutic recuperation, considerations I shall sketch in a moment. The reading I am going to propose is by no means a deconstruction; at best, it will suggest the courses I think a deconstructive reading would need to pursue. I shall be reading texts generally accounted to be "philosophical," whatever that might mean; as such, these texts are admittedly difficult, elitist, and even arcane. Here, I would simply note, following Gramsci, that we are all philosophers: more than philosophy is at stake when it is "philosophy" that is at stake.

In this reading, I am trying to work toward the possibility of a serious and consequent interrogation of the relation between Nishida-philosophy, the thinking of twentieth-century Japan's foremost philosopher, Nishida Kitarō (1870–1945), and the ideological construction of the Japanese state, the so-called emperor-system (*tennōsei*), an investigation that bears directly upon the reading of Ōta Yōko's *City of Corpses*, and thereby upon a consideration of historicity, in Chapter 3. Ostensibly, three issues are at stake. The first is Nishida's personal complicity and involvement in the formulation, "philosophical" authorization, and promulgation of the ideological constructs and propaganda that would presumptively justify the policies of the wartime Japanese government. Were we to pursue this question, we would of course be caught up in the issues of an extensive and repressive censorship, the threat of physical coercion, and the slightly more subtle intimidation by his students, and in questions regarding Nishida's personal naiveté, courage, or mendacity. But such a line of questioning is blocked for us, not only by specific historical circumstances, such as censorship and the existence of the notorious "thought police," but also by the fact that in circumstances such as these, where to speak and to write in many cases meant incarceration and death, one must, I think, presume that a thinker has invested his or her desire and passion in that writing. Under such circumstances, the very division of life from work seems to me to be problematic.

Second, and at least from my perspective more seriously germane, are questions concerning the status of texts produced by Nishida Kitarō for discrete occasions between 1938 and 1945. These texts were addressed to different audiences—philosophy students at Kyoto Imperial University, readers of his philosophical essays, a government-affiliated think tank known as the National Policy Research Association (Kokukaku kenkyūkai) and, indeed, the Shōwa emperor himself.[18] These essays are fundamentally involved with the central terms and slogans of state propaganda and ideology: the *ie* (the "house," *domus*, or family as the organizing principle of the Japanese ethnos), the *kazoku-kokka* (the "family-state," the Japanese state as comprehensive ie), the *minzoku* (*Volk*, people, or race), *kōdō* (the "Imperial Way"), the *kokutai* (the celebrated mystical corporate and corporeal unity of the Japanese state), Japan's "world-historical mission," the "Greater East Asian Co-Prosperity Sphere," the "New World Order," a phrase as bitterly ironic in the 1940's as it is in the 1990's, and *hakkō-ichiū* (the "eight corners of the world under one roof," the dominant slogan of wartime Japanese imperialism, which the leading Japanese-English dictionary persists even today in rendering as "universal brotherhood"). It might be possible to argue that these essays in toto are necessarily cynical effects of an all too certain political exigency. Perhaps: in view of the fact that Nishida died in June 1945, we shall never know.

But, third, it is *also* necessary to take up as the most serious of possibilities for any consideration of Nishida-philosophy, as well as for our own thinking and practice, the possibility that these texts are, in fact, no more and no less than the most explicitly political expressions and articulations of Nishida-philosophy itself, that these texts are in some sense—perhaps in *every* sense—the necessary consequence, the telos, the *meaning* of Nishida-philosophy. And this question must be approached on at least two levels: in terms of their essential continuity with 'Nishida-philosophy' construed as a coherent and systematic formulation of theses, statements, positions, concepts, and "insights" (a conception of 'Nishida-philosophy' that is at least problematic and quite possibly entirely untenable); but also in terms of the *practice* of 'Nishida-philosophy' as a certain kind of textual operation, as a way—or the Way—of thinking itself. This last possibility, that the very movement of a thinking necessarily moves toward *what* was thought in the thinking of these problematic essays, is of course the most dangerous of possibilities; it is also, and *therefore*, a possibility upon which no responsible summary judgment is yet possible, for much remains to be thought. Later I shall try to suggest what is at stake here and suggest something of the investigations that would have to be undertaken to take this possibility seriously. But first, I shall attempt to sketch, however crudely and schematically, the logic of the tennōsei that informs these late political statements, which read the logic of the emperor-system *against* much of contemporary state-sponsored propaganda, but that are thereby all the more dangerous.

In these late political statements, Nishida was clearly concerned to criticize the more blatantly racist formulations of official propaganda. Typically, such formulations tended to ground Japanese claims to hegemony in Asia and the world in the conjunction of biology and cosmology: the Japanese state was seen as a corporate polity (*kokutai*) that was at once a putatively biological essence and the formal expression thereof, at once the essentially genetic and biological continuity of a genealogy (the "house" or ie) with the Volk and with the "family-state." At the same time, the very emperor who was proclaimed to be the head or father of the "family," Volk, and state (entities that thereby become *virtually* identical) was said to be a transcendent deity, a "living god" descended from the sun goddess, Amaterasu. Although few, if any, Japanese took this cosmo-biology very seriously on a literal level, it was undoubtedly taken very seriously indeed as the *mythic* expression of an essential racial superiority, of which the existing Japanese state was the natural and organic form.[19] We know very well, of course, that as both myth and "science," as either myth or "science," this cosmo-biology was taken to authorize Japanese domination—under the banner of "the eight corners of the world under one roof"—as the most banal and brutal of nationalisms. Nishida undertook to criticize the assumption of an unproblematic continuity and essential identity among the "biologically" grounded genealogical "house" or family, the Volk, and the corporate state. Thereby he attempted further to criticize a "mere nationalism," from which nothing other than imperialism, domination, and exploitation could issue. In reworking the defining vocabulary and concepts of official propaganda, he attempted to articulate a vision of a pluralist "world" as a nonsovereign sociality, that is, a world whose order would not be grounded in the threat of violence—in other words, the "eight corners of the

world under one roof" as a humanitarian humanism. To do so was
not only to lend philosophical credence and authority to the most
cynical of official slogans; conversely, it was also, and only *perhaps*
unwittingly, to reveal the violence that is occluded by, but that is
the ultimate authority of, every liberal pluralist humanism.⟩

Nishida repeatedly refused to view the Volk as a preternatural
extension of the family. He took issue, for example, with one Maki
Kenji's "theory of the Japanese corporate polity," which, on
Nishida's account, posited family, family-state, and polity as a corporate collectivity (*dantai*) essentially characterized as (1) natural,
and therefore not an effect of human action, in its constitution and
growth, (2) structurally organized around a center, (3) entirely am-
icable and "friendly" (and therefore with neither difference nor
conflict) in its internal relations and life-activity, and (4) enduring
into the future in an unbroken continuity. A state needs law, Maki
conceded, but in a family-state the morality immanent in the family is the very legality of the law, a morality of which the law as
such is only the actualization; thus, the legal state seeks only to ac-
tualize the life-activity of the corporate community. After an entirely formulaic concurrence with Maki's thesis, Nishida insisted
that the Volk was constituted and formed within and by history and
culture rather than in the biologically determined necessity of nature, and that it therefore surpasses those biological determinations.
The Volk is constituted in the self-consciousness of history and culture, in consciously recognizing itself to *be* in fact a Volk, that is to
say—in ancestor-worship, for example. It is in that self-consciousness, rather than in the "biological" family, the morality that is the
ground of the law comes into being. In self-consciousness, which is
the very distance of self-objectification that separates the historico-
cultural Volk from an unreflective nature, the Volk transcends biology. The corporate polity and the imperium therefore belong to an
essentially different dimension than the family. The emperor is not
immediately the acting *Volkisch* subject; rather, he is that subjectivity's subjectivity, the *ground* of Volkisch subjectivity—and in that
very abstraction, we might add (although Nishida did not), the
"symbol" of the corporate polity. (I might note parenthetically that

Nishida was thereby, as it turned out, theorizing the *postwar* Japanese emperor-system.) But in any case, clearly a certain discontinuity has been introduced into a series that posited the equivalence (or even identity) of family, Volk, state, world, and imperium.[20]

The Volk is coterminous with "history" itself. Indeed, as Nishida instructed the Shōwa emperor, the historical world (as opposed to the natural world, which is not yet an objectified "world" in the strong sense of the word) finds its origins in the fact that a certain Volk lives in a certain geographical location; the *historical* nature of the Volk is an index of its separation from nature (a cultural achievement; indeed, the achievement that *is* "culture"), and most specifically from the presumptive universality of "nature." A Volk is a Volk only insofar as it is *not* indiscriminate species-being, only insofar as it is situated in the constraints of a specific environment or milieu. Originally (an "origin" Nishida was careful to leave unspecified), isolated cultures of isolated *Völker* lived in a mutually determinative relation with the geophysical "climate": a Volk is subject to a certain range of natural determinations and constraints, but it also works on and changes the circumambient milieu, a "work" that is its "cultural" activity. In distancing itself from the presumptively total and irrecusable determinations of nature, it begins the process of producing itself as the active subject that *makes* history. Thus, a Volk is the "force that gives form" to the specifically historical "world" in its very specificity; *in* doing so, it knows itself to do what in fact it does; it achieves a certain level of self-consciousness, and because it is thus the active subject that *makes* history, it belongs to the "creative world." But in the isolation of its mutually determinative cultural relation *with* and *against* nature, a Volk does not yet inhabit a "world." In other words, a Volk-society is not yet a *state.*

In order for a Volk truly to come to self-consciousness (and thus avoid solipsism), truly to know what it in fact (putatively) *is*, it must come into contact and communication with other Völker, it must differentiate itself from what it is *not* and know itself in its difference from others. In that differentiation a "world," and hence "world-history" as the totality that subsumes both self and other in their difference, appears. Various Völker enter into a single "world," a single milieu, which inevitable implies (temporary) rivalry, discord, and war; but also, the amalgamation and unification of various cultures—resulting in a truly "human culture" (Nishida's example was the Roman empire). Today, Nishida told the emperor, the entire globe has become a "world," and contemporary nationalisms must be rethought from such a global perspective. In its encounter with the "world" and its consequent coming to self-consciousness, a Volk necessarily represents itself *to* itself *as* itself. A work of culture, this process is that by which a Volk becomes a *state.*

This process whereby a Volk comes to represent itself as itself, a work of culture in which the state is precipitated, is first of all the work of myth, both the work myth *does* and the work myth *creates.* Myth is not merely the dream of primitive man, Nishida wrote; rather, it is variously the "*form* of the self-formation of a constructed historical society," the "configuration of social production," the "mode of actual life-activity." As such, myth is the image according to which society produces and reproduces itself, is rationalized and individuated. In this movement from myth to reason to individuality, the Volk becomes a state. In other words, myth—the image a given *socius* has of itself and according to which it continually (re)produces itself and *thereby* knows itself to be its self—is what later writers were to call the "social Imaginary." In the case of the Japanese Volk, of course, the dominant myth according to which the corporate polity, of which the state is—precisely—the expression, (re)produces itself is that of the imperium. The imperium is, in fact, the *image* of the very process of imaginary (re)production philosophy has come to call *ekstasis*:

> In the history of our country, the totality is not in opposition to the individual, the individual is not in opposition to the totality; [rather], individual and totality mutually negate each other and, centered upon the imperium, have developed in a vital way. In time, the force of the totality has become something like a center, but it has always been a return yet again to the spirit of the founding of the country; centered upon the imperium, it has crossed yet again into a new epoch, creating that new epoch. Again, history is always moving centered

upon an absolute present that subsumes past and future, but I think that in our country it is the imperium that possesses the significance of an absolute present that subsumes past and future. Therefore I think that to return to the spirit of the founding of our country is not merely to return to the past; it is always again to cross a threshold into a new epoch. Restoration [*fukkō*] is always renovation [*ishin*].[21]

The imperium (and therefore the state of which it is the mythic expression) is therefore identified *both* as the site of an ek-static historical change and (re)productivity (a kind of zero-degree history, or what Nishida called "historical space"), *and* as that which mediates between totality and individual. The totality is nowhere outside of its immanence *in* the individual (and is negated *as* totality precisely because it is immanent *in* and mediated *by* the individual); conversely, the individual *is* an individual only insofar as it *is* the *negation of* the totality. But insofar as the individual is the "negation of" the totality, it is ultimately negated *as* individual and recuperated within the totality. A difficult logic to be sure, and one to which Nishida had devoted vast stretches of philosophical exposition. There can be no question of a discussion here even remotely adequate to the thinking of this thought of what Nishida called "absolute contradictory self-identity" (*zettai mujunteki jikō dōitsu*).[22]

What *is* important for us to consider here is that it is according to this logic in which temporality and sociality converge that Nishida situates the state as the creator of morality and value, as the locus of self-consciousness and the personal in its social relationality, as that which mediates and *resolves* both class struggle and national conflicts, and as the truest expression of the "world-historical mission" of the Volk as creator of the "new world order" signified by the slogan "the eight corners of the world under one roof." Here it will only be possible briefly to mention a few of what Nishida saw as the implications of this logic for politics.

First, the state in no instance merely protects cultural and moral value; on the contrary, the state is that which produces/reproduces value. The state is that which *creates* values (and value itself) because it is essentially the Volk's coming to self-consciousness of its being-in-a-world. The Volk comes to such self-consciousness in and by (re)producing its myths and its inaugural mythos, its material culture, its language and social relations—in short, because it represents itself *to* itself *as* itself in the social Imaginary. And the state, which *is* this jubilant specular self-recognition (*fort-da*?), is also the recognition of the difference between the Volkisch self and others, the demarcation of inside from outside, the *limit* of the self in relation to the Absolute. The state is therefore precisely that which creates morality and value because *as self-consciousness* it *limits*—orders and organizes—the literally anarchic and chaotic (or "prepredicative") possibilities of zero-degree history (i.e., revolution) and zero-degree sociality (the radical singularity of the empirical as such). Furthermore, the state is in fact that limit itself: the imperium, it will be recalled, is the site of zero-degree history. The state is, in other words, the limit that bridges the difference between every order of value and the lawlessness of nonvalue; as such, it *decides* the difference (and does so by sustaining its self—the subjectivity of the Volk—in the [re]productions of the specular Imaginary). Inasmuch as it is self-consciousness of its being-in-a-world, inasmuch as it is a *state*, the Volk takes up the burden of its world-historical mission. I shall return to this point.

Second, because the state is at once the locus and creator of value, it is also that which resolves all conflicts (class struggle, for example), and does so through a reading of "absolute contradictory self-identity" as what has been called a "logic of integration." Recall that the particular and the universal, the individual and the totality, are said *mutually* to negate each other. But in these texts, at least, it is precisely the symmetry of the opposition that privileges the universal or totality, and that because the particular individual is such only as the "negation of" the totality; thus, insofar as the totality negates the individual, the totality merely negates the "negation of" itself. The terms are not convertible; if they were, the totally could only be *virtual*, and one cannot equate a virtual totality with the totality that is the self-consciousness of the Volk's being-in-a-world. In other words, the individual can be the negation of the totality of national self-consciousness only in order to be reintegrated with the totality in the negation of the individual-as-negation-of, suggesting

that the particular individual achieves integration with totality—
and its identity as a member of the Volk—only in the death of the
individual *as* individual. Which is, of course, the promise held out
by the emperor-system as the ultimate integration of the individual in the communal identity of the Volkisch state. Such, indeed,
is the salvation held out to abjection by every humanism, for what
is promised here is the erasure of all difference in the nonexclusive
sociality of the totality, be it Volk or "Man"; what is occluded here
is the violence that in fact installs the abject in abjection.

Were this the extent of Nishida's explicitly political meditations,
had he "concluded" with a valorization, however complex in its
sophistications, of the nation-state as the telos of historical and social
being, his reflections would hold a merely antiquarian fascination
for us. However securely justifications of the nation-state may hold
great numbers of people in their ideological grip, however brutal
the specific material consequences of such nationalisms are still prov-
ing to be, we are, perhaps too easily, persuaded that it is possible to
objectify, and therefore in some way to distance ourselves from, such
formulations. It is therefore *apparently* a relatively straightforward
matter to make a critical judgment, from our presumptively more
nearly enlightened perspective, upon such formulations. But Nishida
went on to criticize such "national egoisms" and attempted, through
a reworking of the significance of current slogans, to envision a
"New World Order" as a pluralist, nonsovereign, global oecumene.
The danger here is not only that such a vision, when articulated in
the terms of the dominant ideology, masks a very real violence and
brutality; but also that such visions harbor within themselves, albeit
"unconsciously," a violence no less terrifying than the most oppres-
sive of nationalisms. It is to this vision, particularly as articulated in
Nishida's address to the National Policy Research Association on
the "fundamental principles of the New World Order," that I shall
—lastly—attend.

Nishida's address opens with a schematic characterization of
successive epochs as apparently essential totalities. The (European)
eighteenth century is characterized as the great age of individualism
and liberalism; nation-states did not yet therefore confront one an-

other in "a single historical world"—England controlled the seas, France the continent. The nineteenth century, however, witnessed belligerent confrontations of nation-states—France, Germany, England—in a "global space," circumstances that led to World War I. The nineteenth century, therefore, was the age of the "self-awareness of the state," of class conflict and of imperialism; there was not yet a *"self-awareness of the world-historical mission of the state"* (Nishida's emphasis). In other words, various European Völker had achieved self-consciousness of their being-in-a-world, but not yet a self-awareness of their being-in-*the*-world; thus the only possible internationalism—communism—was essentially a mere reaction of the "eighteenth century" against the nineteenth. The twentieth century, in the wake of World War I, was the age in which each state had to take up its particular world-historical mission in order to create a *"world-historical world, that is, a global world."* That project was, however, incomplete; the present war would decide the issue.[23]

In order to reach at least an inchoate understanding of what Nishida might have meant by the "world-historical," a "global world," and the "New World Order," it is perhaps worth quoting the text at some length:

> As an effect of the development of the sciences, technology, and the economy, each national Volk has entered a single compact global space. The way to the resolution of this [situation] lies nowhere outside of constructing a single global world by each [national Volk] becoming aware of its own historical mission and, while remaining utterly itself, transcending itself. I therefore call the present age the age of the global self-awareness of each national Volk. To speak of each national Volk transcending itself, thereby constructing one world, is not to speak of the so-called self-determination of Völker as something like recognizing the independence of each Volk equally after the fashion of Wilson's League of Nations. Such a world is no more than an eighteenth-century abstract world-principle. The present world war clearly demonstrates the impossibility of resolving actual problems on the basis of such principles. In that any and every national Volk whatever is established on various historical bases and possesses various historical missions, each national Volk possesses its own historical mission. To say that each national Volk constructs a single

global world by transcending itself while remaining itself means that it
must first of all construct a single particular world *by following its respective regional traditions.* Thus, it is by uniting a particular world on
such a historical basis that the entire world is constructed in a single
global world. In such a global world, each national Volk both lives in
its own individual historical mission, and through its respective world-
historical mission is united in a single global world. This is the furthest
reach of man's historical development; moreover, it is the fundamental principle of the new world order being pursued in the current
world war. Our country's principle of "the eight corners of the world
under one roof" is something like this. . . .

If the problem of the current world war is something on this order, and the fundamental principles of the new world order are posited as above, then the fundamental principles of the [Greater] East
Asian Co-Prosperity Sphere must themselves be derived therefrom.
Thus far, the East Asian Völker have been subjugated, colonized, and
dispossessed of each of their world-historical missions for the sake of
the imperialisms of the European Völker. Today, indeed, the various
Völker of East Asia must become self-aware of the world-historical
missions of the East Asian Völker, and in each transcending itself construct a single particular world, thereby accomplishing the world-historical mission of the East Asian Völker. This is the fundamental principle of the construction of the East Asian Co-Prosperity Sphere. Today, indeed, we East Asian Völker must be aroused world historically,
bearing with us the principles of East Asian culture. But in order for
what we call a single particular world to be constructed, there must be
that which will become the center and stand bearing the burden of
the [world-historical] problem. In East Asia, that is none other than
our Japan. Just as in ancient times the Greek victory in the Persian
Wars determined the direction of the culture of the European world,
so too will the current East Asian war determine one direction in the
world history of later ages.

Today's global morality is neither Christian humanitarianism nor
something on the order of ancient China's "Kingly Way." It is necessarily to speak of each national Volk transcending itself and forming a
single global world; it is necessarily to speak of becoming the architect
of a global world. Our corporate polity is no mere holism [or "to-
talitarianism": *zentaishugi*]. The imperium is the alpha and omega of
our world. The splendor of our corporate polity, enduring for ten
thousand ages, resides in having given form to a single historical world

centered upon the imperium. Our country's imperium is not merely the center of a single Volkisch state. The principle of world-formation, "the eight corners of the world under one roof," is subsumed within the Imperial Way of our country.[24]

the science of monstrosities

Certain "problems," as terrible as those of any teratology, as obscure and as clear as history's own night, are obvious. We are undoubtedly obligated to do more than ponder the nature of the "transcendence" enforced upon other Asians in the process of constituting an East Asian cultural oecumene. And certainly there is sufficient reason for despair at the "New World Order" invoked here, as more recently. It is furthermore undoubtedly legitimate and indeed necessary to ask if the invocations of a "global world" or "world history" are anything other than the sophistications of a certain casuistry, alibis for the most brutal and violent—albeit "transcendent"—domination. (One might well ask, of course, whether every appeal to History is not guilty of the same casuistry.) But it is also necessary to recognize that, in spite of his avowed distance from eighteenth-century cosmopolitanism, Christian humanism, and the League of Nations, Nishida's appeals to the transcendence of world history, of "Man," of the imperium, and of the Co-Prosperity Sphere are in fact appeals to a transcendent universality and a "logic of integration" that are part and parcel of a specifically modern historicist humanism. In arguing that every Volk is possessed of a world-historical mission, and most specifically that every East Asian's mission is to throw off the yoke of Western imperialisms under Japanese leadership, he was holding out the promise of redemption *within* world history to those who had been damned *by* world history to a hell that needed no imagining. In the most brutal terms: you die, but insofar as you die a world-historical death, your death is redeemed by the meaning of world history, your being-in-*the*-world achieves identity. In your particularity, you are the negation of universal world history (or the imperium); but, because as particularity you are the "negation of" universal world history (or the imperium), your "world-historical" fate is to be "negated" *by* the universal; but as negated "negation of" you are recuperated *into* the

totality of a universal world history (or the imperium). It is not for
nothing that the abject sinner, precisely *in* abjection, is promised
redemption by divine grace.

Hegelian? Well, yes, most decidedly. But to notice that the logic
of these texts bears a certain relation to certain possible readings of
Hegel's formulations must lead to a definite and difficult questioning if it is not to remain an observation germane merely to an essentially antiquarian conception of intellectual history as the tracing
of "influences" and the establishment of more or less irrelevant
"comparative" relationships. If the relation to "Hegel" is important, it is important only insofar as that relation is the index of a relation to the teleologies of modern historicist anthropocentrism.
Furthermore, we must ask whether conversely, to the extent that
these political statements are implicated in that teleology, the political consequence of modern historicist anthropocentrism is not expressed in these texts. Bluntly: is the telos and truth of modern humanism to be found precisely at Shanghai and Nanking, Hiroshima
and Nagasaki, Auschwitz and My Lai? Are these events, and a thousand others, merely accidents, unfortunate recidivist barbarisms? We
must at least admit the *question*, for far more than Nishida-philosophy or Hegel are at stake when it is "Nishida-philosophy" or "Hegel" that is at stake.

My point is this: the logic of integration constitutes to a very
large extent the common sense, the unexamined or unthought and
therefore largely unconscious presuppositions of our own thinking;
as such, it informs not only liberal pluralist historicist humanism,
but the historicist humanism of much twentieth-century radical
thought as well—that of György Lukács and of what used to be
called the New Left, for example (in other words, Hegelian Marx-
ism). Precisely because this common sense (common sense both as
a shared set of unexamined assumptions *and* as a self-consciousness
of community—*sensus communis*) constitutes an onto-epistemology,
liberal pluralist historicist humanism and Marxist historicist humanism alike are, entirely contrary to their *expressed* intentions,
nonetheless complicit with—that is, can offer no effective defense
against—totalitarian fascism. I hasten to add, however, that it is not

as if it were possible for any of us unproblematically to reject, or to declare ourselves to be outside of, historicist humanism, whether of the liberal or radical variety: there are no beautiful souls in our histories.

At the risk of redundancy, let me recapitulate what I see to be the main contours of the logic of integration and ask you to consider the extent to which such a logic saturates, as an onto-epistemology, the current situation of the world in which we live, and the extent to which such a logic determines the protocols according to which we live and die. Very schematically, I shall emphasize four points, four points that have been and must be, I think, *targets* for any critical practice oriented toward a future that would be something other than a mere continuity with the present.

(1) There is the assumption that the totality, whether conceived of as God, Man, History, the world, or the imperium, is *immanent* in the individual, that the universal exists nowhere except in its immanence in the particular. In other words, the unity of the totality *is* its dispersion in particularity. But, conversely, this means that the particular is never truly *singular*, because it is always the particular of the universal. Precisely because universalism and particularism are antithetical, they are entirely complicit. It is precisely the *very act* of the particular separating itself from the totality that *expresses* the *essence* of the totality. That movement of absolute separation from the totality by which the individual would declare its own most unique identity is, tautologically, the expression of the identity of the totality.

(2). The destiny or fate of such a particular individual is to be reunited with the totality. The *meaning* of its being is achieved in the transcendence of History-as-totality. The sinner, who in sinning declared his or her particularity, is destined to be reunited with God, the subaltern is reintegrated in the siblinghood of persons (to rewrite Schiller), to achieve its meaning in the communion of human community. But this hermeneutic reunion or reintegration with the totality, this restored plenitude, this recovery of a kind of communitarian amniotic *jouissance*, is accomplished at a price. And that price is always death, the death of the particular *in* its particu-

larity. And that death is a *sacrifice*. The community of the totality is
achieved in the voluntary sacrifice of individuality. This is the promise, and the price, of every patriotism. But it is also the price exacted
for every identification with a community, most particularly that of
Anglo-American liberalism.

   3. This identification, this identity, is achieved in community
construed as a community of the Same. The achievement of this
kind of community, and let us hope there might be other kinds, is
accomplished through what philosophy calls "intersubjective recognition." One presumptively recognizes a preternatural similitude in
another person, and on that basis establishes community through
the communion of communication. But this *assumes* that essential
sameness (that participation in the self-dispersion—one is tempted
to say onanism—of the totality) is *ontological* (in the usual sense of
the term); in other words, there is the assumption that community
is *discovered*. The *discovery* of community construed as an essential
sameness (which is to say, a coming to self-consciousness, the self-
recognition of the community that is supposedly merely the external expression in the "for-itself" of an already existing "in-itself"),
is the *work* of culture—*Einbildungskraft*. Supposedly, as I say, this is
the discovery of an identity that was already there, much as after
the discovery of gravity we suppose that those who lived not
"knowing" gravity nevertheless lived in a gravitational field. And
in this putative "discovery" of communal identity, in this putative
coming-to-self-consciousness in and through representation, historiography has played a central role (as Friedrich Meinecke, for example, knew very well).[25]

   4. The State, as the *nation*-state, is claimed to be the *rationalized expression* of that self-consciousness. In its institutional and constitutional legality, the state claims to be the *ratio* that institutes and
constitutes the identity of the community as such. The Law becomes the logos of being. The State admits of no outside of rationalized being, and claims thereby to be the ultimate horizon of social being. The State claims both to *express*, and in expressing to *be*,
the very identity of the *ethnos*; the State claims to be the identity of
the in-itself and the for-itself precisely because the State bridges the

gap between disorder and order. In a sense, then, the State claims its own status to be, not merely ontological, but the necessary condition of possibility for any ontology. Undoubtedly, it is for this reason that specific governments—which have something to do with what I am calling the State, even if they are not "the State"—are "interested in" the representation of history, which is to say in the mythical and Imaginary constitution of community. The State, which is the institutional and constitutional expression of totality, can tolerate "diversity" only if "diversity" obligates itself to an eventual reunion or reintegration with the totality. The subaltern belongs to History only on condition that he and/or she admits that he and/or she does not really exist.

Now it would require a very long exposition indeed to demonstrate effectively that these four aspects of the logic of integration are necessarily interrelated. I would note in passing, however, that that demonstration has been under way for many years now. But were such a demonstration to be persuasive—and I think it has been—it would mean that there would be no secure place, least of all the place of the historian, from which we could pass judgment on totalitarian fascism, steadfast in our knowledge that our own discourse—indeed, our very denunciation—does not contribute to what has been called the "gathering" of fascism. Let me try to be clear here. I am not saying that we should refrain from denouncing totalitarian fascism in the historical forms in which we have found it; nor am I saying that we are all, somehow, "really" or "secretly" fascists. I am not saying that historicist humanism, whether of the liberal pluralist construction or that of a certain reading of Marx, is somehow really fascism in drag. What I *am* saying is this: totalitarian fascism, with all its horrors, is not a teratological exception to historicist humanism, a kind of bloody syncopation in the rhythm of modernity; it is in fact, *one* of the possibilities of modern humanism. Modern historicist humanism is the condition of possibility for totalitarian fascism, and as such belongs to the gathering of fascism. Fascism cannot, therefore, merely be relegated to the past; it is not merely one historical object among others. Totalitarian fascism is *one* of the possibilities, in some respects already actualized, of the current situation. We cannot, therefore, assume our own thinking and our own work to be "outside" of fascism, or that our own practice is *necessarily* antitotalitarian, simply because we seriously hate fascism, or even because we explicitly reject one or more elements of the logic of integration. (We cannot simply ditch the concept of "totality" and retain our commonsense notions of community and identity, because our commonsense notions of community and identity *necessarily* imply totality.) And so on and so forth. Above all, we cannot simply ditch concepts of totality, particularity, community, identity, and the State and yet leave our commonsense assumptions about historical consciousness and History intact, for these assumptions not only imply a logic of integration, however anti- or non-Hegelian we may proclaim ourselves to be, but historiographical practice too often, and willy-nilly, as the mythology of *Einbildung*, contributes to a politics that we are most committed to reject.

Any practice oriented toward a future that would be something other than a simple continuity with a current situation that includes among its possibilities that of totalitarian fascism must interrogate, in the most radical possible way, those onto-epistemological assumptions that are that practice's ownmost conditions of possibility. And this interrogation is the work of theory. In order to call into question the onto-epistemological conditions of possibility of one's "own" practice, in order to "do" theory, one must specify those conditions of possibility to be *aporiae*, and the investigation of those conditions of possibility to be an "aporetics." (Here, I use the term "aporia," not in its dictionary sense of "doubt," but in the sense in which it is not uncommonly used in philosophy. An aporia in this latter sense means a question that cannot be answered according to the epistemological protocols according to which the question was posed. An aporia, then, specifies a *limit*. To ask, for example, "Why is there history rather than nothing?" leads inexorably to an aporia. In this case, an aporia is both the limit of, and the sole condition of possibility for, what is called historical consciousness. In other words, what makes it possible to speak *as a historian*?)

It is of the very first importance to insist that this practice of aporetics, this ethico-political practice of interrogating the conditions of possibility of one's own thinking, this *theoretical* labor, this labor that *is* "theory," does not, cannot, and must not produce a "new" theory of practice or of history such as would adequately explain and comprehend practice, history, and the world. Just as there can be no general theory of practice, neither can there be a general theory of history. I am, that is to say, talking about a specific response to a specific historical, and specifically *historical*, situation; I am not prescribing a new heaven, a new earth, a new history. For if our enabling aporiae are history's *aporiae*, they are also *history's* aporiae; these aporiae *belong to* history. In other words, the theoretical labor of aporetics or radical interrogation of the conditions of possibility of historical consciousness consists of a *radical historicization*.

Allow me recourse to a few passages from Gramsci in order to try to make myself clear. The first passage occurs late in his critique of Nikolai Bukharin's *Theory of Historical Materialism: A Popular Manual of Marxist Sociology*:

> It has been forgotten that in the case of a very common expression [historical materialism] one should put the accent on the first term— "historical"—and not on the second, which is of metaphysical origin. The philosophy of praxis is absolute "historicism," the absolute secularization and earthliness of thought, an absolute humanism of history. It is along this line that one must trace the thread of the new conception of the world.[26]

I note, not at all in passing, that this is very much part of a critique of what we now call in a certain shorthand the "metaphysics of presence." But one might begin to read this passage by asking, What differentiates an "*absolute* historicism," which would be a Marxist historicism, from garden-variety historicism (and it is fairly clear that Gramsci never forgets Croce's idealist historicism)? We might approach this question from the perspective of two other citations, drawn from a discussion of the "historicity of the philosophy of praxis":

> [E]ven the philosophy of praxis is an expression of historical contradictions, and indeed their most complete, because most conscious,

expression; this means that it too is tied to "necessity" and not to a "freedom" which does not exist and, historically, cannot yet exist. If, therefore, it is demonstrated that contradictions will disappear, it is also demonstrated implicitly that the philosophy of praxis too will disappear, or be superseded. In the reign of "freedom" thought and ideas can no longer be born on the terrain of contradictions and the necessity of struggle. At the present time, the philosopher—the philosopher of praxis—can only make this generic affirmation and can go no further; he cannot escape from the present field of contradictions, he cannot affirm, other than generically, a world without contradictions, without immediately creating a utopia. . . .

. . . If the philosophy of praxis affirms theoretically that every "truth" believed to be eternal and absolute has had practical origins and has represented a "provisional" value (historicity of every conception of the world and of life), it is still very difficult to make people grasp "practically" that such an interpretation is valid also for the philosophy of praxis itself, without in so doing shaking the convictions that are necessary for action.[27]

Reading them over the past few years, I have found these passages extraordinarily provocative in many respects and at many levels—personal, professional, political. And I have not really even begun to think what their resonance might be in terms of an integral reading of Gramsci, or what their implications might be for any consideration of Gramscian politics. At the moment I simply want to indicate several aspects of these passages that are germane to the present discussion. First, and quite obviously, they were produced, as we know, in a "current situation" in which the "question" of totalitarian fascism was more than a possibility, and concomitantly that Gramsci's interest in the "question of practice," as an orientation toward a future that would be something other than a continuity with the present, was more than speculative. Second, these passages resonate very strongly with thousands of pages of Nishida's work that I have not discussed here but that contradict, often quite explicitly, the formulations of the texts I *have* presented. In this respect, it is impossible to come to a straightforward judgment on either Nishida or Gramsci, precisely because any responsible reading of these texts finds its own enabling assumptions in question. Third, because such texts explicitly, or so it seems to me, propose a relation to conceptions of historicity and community rather different from the currently hegemonic conceptions of history, identity, and society.

Here, it seems to me, Gramsci is not only attempting to think a "philosophy *of* praxis" as the theoretical ground of practice; he is also attempting to think a philosophy of praxis to be *itself* a practice "on the terrain of contradictions and the necessity of struggle." Thus, "historical consciousness" must be thought to be theoretically and practically productive only to the extent that it is recognized to be a contradiction. Historical consciousness is at once the consciousness *of* history, the capacity to posit that "there is history rather than nothing," and a consciousness that is itself specifically historical, an effect of, and subject to, the vicissitudes of history. Insofar as historical consciousness posits the "existence" of history, it must posit itself as a rationality to which past and future alike are essentially comprehensible. The present is a fundamentally rational effect of the past, the future a fundamentally rational effect of our acting in the present. The future, albeit the field of a certain limited indeterminacy, in its fundamental rationality defines acting in the present to be a no less rational project, oriented toward a specific future, a utopia. In this case, historical consciousness is that which takes history to be an object for consciousness and thereby claims to know its object. Thus, it necessarily situates itself as an essentially positive knowing *outside* of history; history is thereby no longer the ultimate horizon of being.

But if "historical consciousness" is to be that which enables political acting in the present, it cannot abstract itself from the "present field of contradictions." Therefore, "historical consciousness" must also be the acknowledgment of its own nontranscendence. In order to enable—or to *be*—a practice or praxis in the current situation, historical consciousness must undertake to think its own radical contingency, its historicity; it must think futurity (for Marx and Gramsci alike, "communism," what Gramsci called an "*absolute* humanism") to be the site of historical consciousness's own "disappearance," extinction, or "supersession," the limit of its epistemological and practical possibilities. In this sense, historical consciousness is the guarantee of the encounter of the philosopher of praxis (or historian) with the radical difference that "is" futurity: communism is not a rational project, because its mode is that of discontinuity. The contradiction of the historical consciousness of *any* philosophy of praxis is that it must think history to be both transcendence and the guarantee of nontranscendence, continuity and discontinuity, ideality and materiality, knowing and its other. And it must do so precisely in order to situate itself as a political (which is to say, nonneutral) practice in the current situation, in order, that is to say, to think its own historicity. In order to *be* a historically determinate practice, it must think its own finitude, its own limit. It is only in its *explicit* refusal to project a utopian, mythological, imaginary community of sameness and identity that a critical practice can assume the burden of its own historicity.

Now this limit, which marks the essential otherness of both past and future, is not merely a boundary between the known and the unknown, between what we know and what we do not yet know but is—ideally—knowable. This limit is the limit of knowability as such, the aporia of historical consciousness. But as essential difference, this aporia, *which resists historicization absolutely*, can only be designated within a discourse entirely bound to historical consciousness, as a radical negativity. We can never say what it is that resists our knowing absolutely; it follows that neither can we *determine* those limits themselves. We can think neither the unthinkable itself nor the determinations of the limits of thinkability. Neither, then, can we merely invoke the aporiae of historical consciousness (as "irrationality") in order to valorize any discourse, practice, or acting whatever.

But if we cannot think, as such, either the outside or the limits of historical consciousness, we can think the thought of the limit. Just as in mathematics, the zero and infinity designate no positive referents but rather the very *impossibility* of designating a positive referent, so too the aporiae of historical consciousness—materiality, the event, communism, for example—designate only the specific impossibilities of referentiality for historical consciousness: *any phi-*

losophy of praxis can think itself as practice only on the condition that it think itself as a thinking the thought of that which is strictly speaking unthinkable. If it fails to do so, it must resign itself to the ahistorical passivity of transcendental subjectivity.

If thinking the thought of the limit of historical consciousness is a necessary condition of possibility, if not guarantee, for thinking any philosophy of praxis to be itself, as critical practice, a praxis, it is such only to the extent that this thinking the thought of the limit is not merely a propaedeutic gesture, but an integral and necessary aspect of that practice itself. Which is to say that critical practice is the "introduction" of an *essentially unassimilable* otherness into our thinking, an explicitly political act in that it is only in the "introduction" of this unassimilability into our thinking that politicality—the possibility totalitarian fascism denies—can be conceived. This politicality is that which opens upon the unassimilability of that which—those who—in resisting the usual courses of historicization absolutely *thereby* resist assimilation and integration absolutely. It is for this reason that the subaltern historiographies to which an increasing number of professional historians are committed imply far more than the proliferation of objects under the panoptic Gaze of the historian. Rather, they insist upon their unassimilable difference at the level of our founding epistemological assumptions. History, whatever it was once thought to be, must be thought as the very impossibility of achieving integration, and historiography as the very impossibility of achieving onto-epistemological consensus.

This is indeed central to what counts for me as deconstruction. It is sometimes objected with regard to such critical practices that they are at best ironic, or at worst, nihilistic. But if we pursue Gramsci's meditation seriously, I have tried to suggest, we must recognize that the historico-social—communism—always surpasses and transgresses the closures of "history," "society," and "identity." And this radical contingency of the historico-social—communism—is itself essential rather than contingent: it is this essential radical contingency or historicity of "communism" that the critical practice of deconstruction, as a philosophy of praxis, honors.[28] To conceive critical practice as a positive project—as "reconstruction," say—

would be to posit—at least ideally, and let us hope *only* ideally—a coherent totality immanent in its dispersions and therefore identical to itself, which would *know* itself to be identical to itself, and which both historically and socially would be functionally integrated, a totality within which critique could only be the fine-tuning of a well-tempered machine—a machine that, like the liberalism of Marx's bourgeoisie, would be without history because it possesses *a* history.

It is only a theoretico-critical practice that can hope to achieve the historical specificity necessary to any critique of fascism, because it is only in the essentially *theoretical* operation of thinking the thought of the limit that our thinking and practice can achieve the nonneutrality of a truly *political* praxis. In this respect, the political task of what I call deconstruction must be carried out between two exigencies, which I mark in closing with two citations. The first is Marx's perhaps too familiar eleventh thesis on Feuerbach: "The [historians] have thus far only interpreted the world: the point, however, is to change it." The second is from Antonio Negri, who knows something about practice himself: "Revolution has hitherto only perfected the state; the point, however, is to destroy it."[29]

CHAPTER 3

Apocalypse Now—Forever—Whenever

Let's face it: we're all in this together, oh gentle reader; and no
one—and that includes you and me, both—gets out of here, alive.

—Sue Golding, "Pariah bodies"

The Apocalyptic Sublime

It has long been commonplace, of course, to encode the events
of 6 and 9 August 1945 in Hiroshima and Nagasaki, the consequent
possibility of nuclear disaster, and the very real presence of nuclear
terror, ecological disasters, and the AIDS pandemic, as apocalyptic
events or as crises that bear within themselves, as their essential possibility, the potential for an apocalyptic actualization. The logic here
is as seductive as it is familiar. In whatever form the apocalypse has
been imagined, or precisely in the impossibility of imagining the
form of the apocalypse, it has been thought as the inescapable sublime coincidence of an unremitting nihilism with a no less unremitting soteriology. The logic of the apocalyptic implies the necessary and simultaneous conjunction of the utter annihilation of
what is with the eschatological revelation of the meaning and truth
of all that has been and is (the historian's long-awaited Götterdämmerung), as well as the transcendence of the apocalyptic event in
the kerygmatic disclosure of that truth and meaning. Indeed, the
logic of the apocalyptic necessarily implies that the annihilation itself of what is must be construed as nothing less than the revelation
of Truth. The utter nihility of the apocalypse is therefore the Truth

of all that has been, might have been, is, might be, or shall be. Thus, that very impossibility of transcendence, the nontranscendence or finitude that would be the very *Ereignis*, the event or occurrence, of the apocalypse, becomes thus the transcendence of its materiality or historicity—as fate, destiny, or classical *devotio*, for example. The apocalypse is thus cast as the seduction of contradiction: nihility is the meaning of all being, death is the Truth of being in an inexorable teleology within which deliverance or salvation is not to be denied. The end of history, as annihilation, becomes the end of history, as telos; the end of history thus becomes the time at the end of time that brings time to an end.

By the terms of this logic, of course, the thought of the apocalypse can only be a figure in the historical Imaginary because the apocalypse can only be situated in the future, always postponed for existing beings. Which makes the apocalypse that which identifies those who envision the apocalyptic to be, in fact, oracular seers or prophets, witnesses to a future that is the end of the very possibility of futurity. The effects of this apocalyptic Imaginary have been traced often enough: to envision the apocalypse makes us of us, here and now, tragic heroes devoted, in the classical sense of the devotio, to that destruction which would be, not only our consolation, but our redemption, our resurrection. But this tragic devotion to the figure of a redemptive apocalypse, this cosmological patriotism, immediately, here and now, denies the very possibility of futurity, of praxis, of what is called agency, of anything, indeed, except the valorization of or acquiescence in the obliteration of possibility itself; we become nothing more, nothing other, than those who will have died, but whose extermination can only be witnessed in the prolepsis of oracular prophecy.[30]

At least in its general configuration and in its more obvious implications, the dangers of the apocalyptic vision are clear enough; and yet, precisely because materially the actualization of one or another apocalypse is entirely within the range of technological possibility, the thought of the apocalypse cannot be abandoned altogether. To do so would be to trivialize, perhaps quite fatally, what must be thought in order to think the thought of nuclear terror, ecological disaster, or AIDS. But the thought of the apocalypse must be thought, perhaps impossibly, without the concomitant thought of redemption or the tragic, a thought that would be sustained by no trope whatsoever. Does the inevitable prolepsis of the thought of any apocalypse, necessarily situated in the future anterior, thereby *necessarily* imply the thought of redemption or resurrection? Can the thought of the apocalypse be figured outside of the oracular or the prophetic? Here let us note that the oracle or prophet who speaks of the past is called quite simply a historian; is it then perhaps that the logic of the apocalyptic brings with it an unbearable fatality, not because its gaze is directed to the future (that history Walter Benjamin's Angelus Novus could not bear to face), but because its logic is that of every invocation of history?

What would be at stake, then, in the thought of the apocalypse would be the thought of the event as absolute and incommensurable difference, historicity as the surplus of conceptuality, materiality in the singularity of its infinite entropic undifferentiated difference as the surplus of ideality: historicity as the thought of the unthinkable, the intuition of the aporetic. Further, such an "event," such historicity, such materiality must necessarily be thought of in respect of historical situation, the historical situation of historicity. Here, "situation" could not designate merely "context," because in its ordinary usages the term "context" implies a certain ready comprehensibility. A situation, a historical situation, designates rather existential exigency itself, the force of an Outside that is not merely the outside of an inside, but the outside that is inside, the insidious inside. Unless one posits that the intuition of the aporia is simply an insight that occurs to transcendental subjectivity, or more crudely, a "stroke of genius," then this intuition of the aporia (that is, the thought of historicity) must be thought as an effect of a certain, even if indeterminable, historical situation. More, it must in some sense designate an "experience," but an experience that is always and necessarily the excess, surplus, impossibility, or *limit* of the phenomenological experience of a subject. The historical situation of historicity must be thought as the "relation" of existential exigency, that exigency which "is" the existential, to historicity. And this relation, so called, necessarily marks a limit for historical consciousness, the aporetic limit-experience that is at once the sole condition of possibility for every historicization but cannot itself be historicized or, indeed, conceptualized, except as the failure, the ruin, the crashing of conceptuality.

In other words, what is at stake here is the intuition of the sheer improbability of the fact "that there is" history, that it is at all possible to ask, "Why is there history rather than nothing?" That there is history can only be intuited within, and as the intuition of, an aporetic historicity, an intuition that is the very impossibility of the intuition of the Kantian a priori of space and time (which is the condition of possibility for every historicization or invocation of the historical). As the exigency that is the existential, this contradiction—the intuition of the aporetic impossibility of the intuition—is not merely a theoretico-philosophical limit, but also the ground of the historico-social and the political altogether. And this means we must attempt to think the historically situated impossibility of historicization. Consequently, what is at stake here is not a relation of correspondence or commensurability between thought and its presumptive object, which would be merely a hermeneutic or epistemological problem, but the question of a nonrelation, a nonrelating relation, the relation that *is* nonrelation. Precisely because what is at issue is the exigency of the existential, the "bite of the Real" as Christopher Fynsk says, the apocalyptic, as the thought of a radical historicity, can never be conceptualized; it can only mark the site or limit of conceptuality. This aporia must be sustained: the thought of the apocalyptic, as the material existentiality that is historicity (or finitude), must be thought as the impossibility or limit for a thought of the apocalyptic. Otherwise, of course, the thought of the apocalypse is merely the prophecy of a sublime utopia.

This means, first of all, if we are to think the apocalyptic as something other than tragic destiny or redemption, that Apocalypse Now must be thought, not as the telos of a historical development, but in its present possibility, its everydayness, in and as that banality of the quotidian which would be at the same time the irremediable interruption of the everyday. Furthermore, the possibility of the apocalyptic must be thought in its irreversibility; whether we are speaking of nuclear terror, ecological disaster, or AIDS, we must recognize the magic bullet, the cure, the solution, to be fantasmatic objects of a nostalgia. Finally, we must acknowledge the radical contingency of the apocalypse, that from the perspective of the experiencing subject of a phenomenology, however informal, the apocalypse is ultimately unpredictable: apocalypse now, forever, whenever. Wherever, whoever, whatever. In short, we must think the apocalyptic as an infinite and indifferent *punctuality*. This punctuality would not be the punctuation that would mark either fate or destiny; neither would it be the punctuation that brings a narrative temporality to term. Punctuality here would indicate, precisely, a nondelay that is not presence, the indifference of the time of material singularity, that entropic "historical space" which would be radical atemporality; what must be thought here is the indifferent, infinite punctuality of the infinite difference of whatever singularities, the very time of AIDS in its contingency, as well as the contingency that makes of the whenever, whatever, forever of nuclear extinction a terrorism.

Now it is my argument that it is the very everydayness of the quotidian, as well as the thematization and valorization of its normative regularities, in which custom becomes nomos, that occludes the apocalyptic that has been, since 6 August 1945, the ground of social and political life. The everyday—which is to say, a "lived relation" or nonrelation to the material conditions of existence—occludes the apocalyptic through the work of culture, through a certain *technē*, a certain construction of the conjunction of use and need (*Brauch*), through the historicization-cum-*Bildung* that is the work of mourning, through the occlusion of a radical absence-of-work (madness, as Foucault would say). But if the everyday is revealed in the ideologicality of its lived relations to be sedimented systems of significations that are taken to be natural in their very occlusion of historicity, it is paradoxically the case that the ground of that very everydayness is precisely that terror, the excess of any possible ontology, that is the possibility of nuclear annihilation, of ecological disaster, and of AIDS. In other words, the specificity of the everyday in the time of nuclear terror, ecological disaster, in the time of AIDS, can only be thought as a nonrelating relation (the relation of occlusion) to the apocalyptic.

In order to pursue this congeries of questions, aporiae, and contradictions, I shall be reading two texts in this and the following chapters: Takenishi Hiroko's "The Rite" ("Gishiki"), first published in 1963, and Ōta Yōko's *City of Corpses* (*Shikabane no machi*), first published in a censored edition in 1948 and reissued in a second, uncensored edition in 1950.[31] I must emphasize that in reading texts of the so-called A-bomb literature or, for that matter, the so-called AIDS literature, my interest lies neither in rendering an aesthetic judgment upon what are called works of art nor in the objectification of such textual practices as documents, as the exemplary objects of a sensibility, epoch, spirit, age, or discourse—"modernity," for example—that could be subjected to the usual courses of historiographical predication, comparativity, narrativity, and judgment; such a project, whatever value it might have, would nevertheless remain securely within the confines of interpretation, knowing, and the understanding, in its aspiration to hermeneutic revelation defined and determined as its distance from, and therefore its relation to, transcendental subjectivity construed as possibility. So it will not be a question of the positivist accuracy of these texts in representing and interpreting the radical incommensurability of that to which they bear witness, nor of my adequacy in deciphering the essential meaning of these texts. Rather, because what is most centrally at stake is the possibility that, insofar as these texts can be read to insist upon the radical unintelligibility of a Real that resists interpretation, the understanding, knowledge, meaning, and the aspiration to transcendental subjectivity absolutely, a Real to which any historiographical teratology, phenomenology, or hermeneutic is necessarily and forever inadequate, such texts, so called, are interventions or provocations—performative rhetorics, or, indeed polemics—that might awaken us from our epistemological lethargies to a serious and consequent encounter with that impossibility for knowing that is at the same time the sole condition of the possibility for knowing, and thereby move us toward something that might be called thinking or acting, independent of the narcotic comforts of an always, in fact, deferred epistemological certitude. My reading, although it is indeed a thematic reading, is an *explication de texte* only to the extent that my guiding question concerns *what is at stake* in these texts. For it is precisely because these texts are profoundly and originally implicated in a nonrelating relation (the relation of nonrelation) to the exigency of the existential, the force of the Outside, that the normative protocols of contextualization and historicization become problematic. The *situation* of Takenishi's and Ōta's writing—the attempt to contextualize, historicize, or simply make sense of the apocalyptic event, as well as the failure and the necessity of that attempt—finds its analogue in any attempt to contextualize and historicize these texts themselves. And this by virtue of the "historical situation" itself, for these texts bear witness to the ultimate impossibility of witnessing; they are testimony to the impossibility of the presence of the event.

The Work of Mourning

The main outlines of the usual courses of the work of mourning are undoubtedly well known. Very schematically, we know that the work of mourning, including mortuary rituals, remembering, and various memorializations, is a process by which the dead are rendered radically *other* by means of a process of dissociation or separation that is simultaneously and thereby a process of objectification, a process whereby a certain "that" is acknowledged to be nothing more than an abject object: dead meat. At once a labor of abjectification and objectification, the work of mourning *historicizes* the dead, and in historicizing the dead restores the wounded ego to its integral propriety; precisely the same labor that must be undertaken, according to Freud's *Beyond the Pleasure Principle*, to overcome, through contextualization, the trauma of the singular, radically contingent event. In any case, in the work of mourning, to relegate the dead to the past is to render the other abject, to expel the object from the realm of the living—a double movement, therefore: both the constitution of a *historical* object (historicization) and

the production of an essentially abject social surplus. To this highly
abstract formulation of the work of mourning, however, I must ap-
pend a number of not entirely miscellaneous observations and draw
a few relatively obvious inferences.

First, I would note that in Freud's first consideration of the
work of mourning, which in the text he calls "recollection,"
mourning is relegated to the margins of daily life, to the leisure of
an avocation, the outside of a certain domesticity.[32] Seemingly, this
successful work of mourning is entirely secondary to the cultural
work of the *domus*, posing no substantial threat to that work. Pursuing the relation of the work of mourning to the domestic work of
culture beyond the Freudian text, we might ask whether that relation is merely incidental. What does the separation (from "nature")
that is the putative accomplishment of culture have to do with separation from the abject dead? Does the work of mourning merely
sustain the work of culture, or is the relation perhaps more complex: is it perhaps that the work of culture is in itself a work of
mourning? How might that relation, if relation there be, be articulated?

Second, I would note that the historicization which is the work
of mourning depends, if it is to be undertaken at all, upon what in
the Freudian vocabulary would be called "reality testing," the witnessing and verification that the corpse is in fact (and in its facticity)
nothing but dead meat, the material, abject residue of a cathected
object. The therapeutic processes of historicization depend upon
the ostensibly empirical procedures of producing an image of what
is called reality.

Third, and concomitantly, this witnessing and verification of
the abjection of the corpse is the condition of possibility for the rituals that in and as their enactment establish and confirm the separation between past and present, presence and absence, life and
death, remembering and repetition; the rite is the nomological enactment of the *fort-da*; what is reenacted in every mortuary ritual is
the originary separation of every binary opposition, the inaugura-
tion of the very possibility of sense and meaning, the institution of
the logos itself. The rite confirms in its every repetition the possi-

bility of a ground for a shared intelligibility. The act of separation performed around that corpse, which is the image of an absolute senselessness, secures for those who perform the ritual the guarantee of a common pathos, a common sense. Thus, the rite is the instauration of community precisely because it separates we the living from the unutterably abject dead. Mourning becomes Bildung, a process continually reenacted, which in its reenactments produces the image of cultural community.

Fourth, the failure of this work of mourning, its incompletion or unachievement, is therefore a pathological melancholia, that open wound or piercing which obviates the possibility for an absolute separation.[33] Whereas in a successfully accomplished work of mourning, the ego is restored to the propriety of its separation from the abject object, in the failure of the work of mourning, the ego fails to reconstitute itself: "In mourning it is the world which has become poor and empty; in melancholia it is the ego itself."[34] Which is to say that in melancholia there is a (narcissistic) "*identification* of the ego with the abandoned object."[35] As with every vampire or ghost, the problem of Rilke's angels, melancholics who "don't always know / if they're moving among / the living or the dead," is that they cannot sustain the logos, the binary that is its support, and thus the community of intelligibility by which we separate ourselves, through a certain occlusion, from our historicity.

That is to say, all of this encodes melancholia and traumatic neurosis as psychological dysfunction, as a disaster that befalls a subject; the melancholic is an ill-fated autonomous ego who is hypercathected on an abject object with which, by definition, the melancholic identifies. These neuroses are therefore constituted in the failure of historicization, in the inability to sustain the nomological, putatively ontologically regulative, binary oppositions of presence and absence, life and death, remembering and repetition; these neuroses are therefore the impossibility of maintaining the preeminently cultural work of mourning, which is a kind of forgetting of destitution and abjection, ultimately a forgetting or occlusion of the traumatic force of that existentiality which, in respect of the ego, is a wound.[36]

But perhaps there is a different way to think all this. Mourning, melancholia, and trauma always refer to something that happens to someone else, to the suffering or loss of others or of objects, or of others as libidinal objects. Mourning, melancholia, and trauma are always occasioned by the historicity of the other, which implies that "our" historicity always comes to "us" as the death of the other. Indeed, we can only mourn ourselves as objects in the proleptic separation from what we take ourselves to "be"; thus, historicity can be "experienced" (as a passage to the limit of what can be phenomenologically experienced) only *as* sociality: *sociality is the very existentiality of historicity*, historicity is therefore never my "ownmost" except as that separation which is the apocalyptic failure of sociality. Furthermore, insofar as the work of mourning reveals sociality to be the very existentiality of historicity, sociality is an originarily asymmetrical relation, a nonrelating relation, the relation of nonrelation, and hence the surplus of every intersubjectivity or psychology: the community of intelligibility and sense is therefore grounded in the very impossibility of communication:

> Now, "the basis of communication" is not necessarily speech, or even the silence that is its foundation and punctuation, but the exposure to death, no longer my own exposure, but someone else's, whose living and closest presence is already the eternal and unbearable absence, an absence that the travail of deepest mourning does not diminish. And it is in life itself that the absence of someone else has to be met. It is with that absence—its uncanny presence, always under the prior threat of a disappearance—that friendship is brought into play and lost at each moment, a relation without relation or without relation other than the incommensurable. . . . Such is, such would be the friendship that discovers the unknown we ourselves are, and the meeting of our own solitude which, precisely, we cannot be alone to experience.[37]

I shall have frequent occasion to return to this passage; indeed, all of Chapters 5 and 7 are in some sense a meditation on this passage. For the present, I shall simply note that it is from here that a thought of a being-in-common bereft of the consolations of modern humanism must proceed.

For, finally, what if the ego, enveloped in the prophylaxis of its armor, together with the intersubjective comforts and consolations that sustain it, is not taken to be ontologically given, but is, rather, an exception to sociality in its originary historicity? What if, that is to say, the cultural consolations—those consolations that constitute culture (through the work of mourning, for example)—that sustain the ego constitute no ground, but are conversely parentheses in the absolute and irremediable destitution of what is? What if, as the history of the twentieth century has confirmed for so many, horror is what used to be called the "human condition"? What if that relation of nonrelation which is the relation to the exigency of the existential is in fact the secret hidden in the most intimate recesses of what we take to be our being? What if Derrida is right when he writes regarding the AIDS pandemic:

> The various forms of this deadly contagion, its spatial and temporal dimensions will from now on deprive us of everything that desire and a rapport to the other could invent to protect the integrity, and thus the inalienable identity of anything like a subject: in its "body," of course, but also even in its entire symbolic organization, the ego and the unconscious, the *subject* in its separateness and in its absolute secrecy. The virus (which belongs neither to life nor to death) may *always already* have broken into any "intersubjective" space. And considering its spatial and temporal dimensions, its structure of relays and delays, no human being is ever safe from AIDS. This possibility is thus installed at the heart of the social bond as intersubjectivity. And at the heart of that which would preserve itself as a dual intersubjectivity it inscribes the mortal and indestructible trace of the third— not the third as the condition for the symbolic and the law, but the third as destructing structuration of the social bond, as social disconnection (*déliaison*) and even as the disconnection of the interruption, of the "without rapport" that can constitute a rapport to the other in its alleged normality.[38]

In the time of nuclear terror, ecological disaster, and of what is called AIDS, any consequent thinking must think itself first of all to be situated within the nontranscendent existentiality of the apocalyptic. In the first instance, this imposes a certain *askēsis* upon us, for this thought of the apocalyptic must be thought neither as despair nor as redemption—nor, for that matter, as celebration. Concomitantly, we must acknowledge the essential impossibility of thinking that absolute resistance which nontranscendence offers to thought, but which nevertheless offers itself to thought, imperatively, as absolute resistance to thought. It is precisely that resistance to thought and the concept which must be thought from within an askēsis, that is the refusal of every consolation. It is from here the we might begin to think the provocations of texts by Takenishi Hiroko and Ōta Yōko.

Unaccomplished Mourning

Takenishi Hiroko's "The Rite" can be read as a meditation on the radical and unavoidable unaccomplishment of the work of mourning, on the very impossibility of undertaking the work of mourning, for "The Rite" is written around "the sudden loss of all I thought was mine," including the propriety of the proper self, "and the omission of the rite that should have been performed" (198–99). We are confronted by Takenishi with the impossibility of that inaugural act which would establish (or, presumptively, reestablish) the regulatory *nomos*, that law of separation which is established only in its transgression. Here, the establishment of a Law of binary opposition (the very possibility of Symbolic order as such) is inaugurated only in the transgression of that Law; thus, the text meditates on the disjunct simultaneity, the coincidence, of both parturition and death.

The text opens upon the scene of an impoverished, domestic funeral, observed by Aki, the protagonist, from the security of the doorway of her own house, the security of the domus before the advent for Aki of historicity; this remains the memory of a fascination "from the far off days of her childhood, long before Aki had ever experienced such things as the sickness or death of her own flesh and blood" (171). For Aki, the events leading to this modest, "poor" rite all occur within a securely established and imperturbable domesticity; the funeral in fact establishes the regularity of the quotidian of which it is a part. Here it is precisely the impoverished ordinariness, the banality of the scene, that is important, for it is precisely as the funerary rite interrupts daily life that it confirms and justifies the Law of the quotidian, its regulatory regularities. This is an entirely nonpathological, successful, and accomplished work of mourning (169–71).

This is followed by one of a series of short scenes, which punctuate the text at irregular intervals, of an adult Aki in an *essential* unease, which is at the same time a kind of essential nostalgia for the securities of the domus (171–72).

There follows yet another scene of an adequate, successful, and above all accomplished mourning; but this time it is a matter of what Michel de Certeau called the "historiographical operation"[39] and the historical Imaginary. Yet again, however, it is a question of fascination—in the first instance a fascination with the *image* of a "young Egyptian nobleman" on the lid of a funerary urn (which held the internal organs) on the cover of a weekly magazine purchased under the Gaze of the others of quotidian life (others who are in fact, however, profoundly inattentive to Aki's fascination). The image on the urn is that of one who has been mummified, one whose image witnesses and certifies that the (un)dead belong to history. Under the image of the face, the image of the presence of an absence, are contained the viscera, which are not part of the image of the body, but are, rather, the scraps of an essentially uncontainable materiality. But the photograph of the image on the funerary urn also bears the weight of a certain exoticism, of an "ancient Egypt" as the object of and for the anthropological, historiographical Gaze. An exoticism that will be repeated and echoed in a catalogue of exotic funeral rites (180), this exoticism will be nuanced not only by the fact that the diplomat husband of Setsuko, a dying friend of Aki's, sends his wife postcards "[f]rom a café terrace that had a view of the Sphynx [*sic*]" (179), but also by the fact that at O-Bon, the Buddhist festival of the revenant, the presence of the dead, Aki will notice the wallpaper, faded but still distinct in its image of the quotidian task of a woman washing a jar in a stream against a background of the Pyramids, the place of the dead fathers (192). Here the historical Imaginary itself is the scene of a consolatory reconciliation, of a successful work of mourning in an accomplished historicization, and thereby of a certain redemption:

> There without a doubt was a fitting way to start out on death's journey, with the dead well tended and watched over by the living. Thinking of that man who had left behind a part of his own flesh, and the people who had taken it into their keeping, in what was surely a most dignified and solemn ceremony, it seemed to Aki that there indeed was a secure and reassuring way to die. (173)

The contemplation of the historical Imaginary constructed in the historiographical operation—an archaeology that disturbs the dead in order, in a virtual exorcism, to lay them like ghosts—is itself the *promise* of solace and redemption. This Imaginary is held out as the promise that history and historicization do not merely mark but are in themselves consolatory and redemptive. For all of this, Aki retains a kind of nostalgic fascination (itself the coincidence, of course, of attraction and repulsion). Indeed, she seeks to position herself, and thus establish the very possibility of "herself," within the nostalgia of that historical Imaginary; she is keenly aware that "identity" is achieved only in assuming an objectness within that Imaginary, in seeing but also in being seen, in being both the Gaze and its object. And yet Aki recognizes that this specular historical identification is for her impossible.

First, her identification is not with the image of the Egyptian, but with the figure of the Jew:

> My ancestors were slaves in Egypt . . . like the people of Israel, who at the Feast of the Passover, yearning to break free from bondage, woke from sleep and resumed reading their dark records. At that time, their thoughts probably ran like this—Someone who can just casually wipe out the memory of his own history will not be fit, as history unfolds, to play the role of a great hero. (199)

Second, her identification is with the figure of a "woman" for whom specular identification in the historiographical Imaginary is essentially traumatic, a recognition that historical science is the "science of the father." Recalling a childhood memory of domestic violence, she wonders,

Why was she upsetting herself over that unknown woman who was undoubtedly cowering on the other side of the garden wall? Aki, still only a child, did not know, but in some obscure hurt way she felt a sense of identity with the woman beyond the wall. Are all women doomed to weep like that when they grow up? . . . Aki felt that she was falling, falling down into a black abyss, and then discovered that she herself was crying. (190)

But Aki's figure of the woman is not of the woman who would be merely the inverse figure of the man, for in what psychoanalysis would diagnose as melancholia (as if diagnosis were the point here), and in response to a certain existentiality, Aki withdraws her libidinal cathexis from her lover Noboru (196). Her principal relations are with other women, Tomiko and Setsuko.

For ten years a classmate of Aki's (and therefore probably, although this is never said explicitly, like Aki, a *hibakusha* [a victim of the bombing]), Tomiko is pregnant for the third time. Her two previous miscarriages were possibly effects of the bombing. In any event, Tomiko is intent upon fulfilling the narrative expectations of a domestic maternity. For Tomiko, the figure of the woman is defined by the coincidence, or indeed identity, of maternity with domesticity; this is not necessarily so for Aki herself. Tomiko regards her pregnancy as the punctuality of a narrative (175), and she reassures herself on this point with the word of her husband. But the comforts held out by this triad—maternity, domesticity, historical narrative—is interrupted by the force of a certain existentiality: miscarriages. In a meditation on funerary urns more essentially disturbing than that of the Egyptian nobleman, within the domestic arrangements of Tomiko's house, Aki notices "two small jars, standing low there side by side and all but buried under the flowers. The fetuses that had miscarried, as if this were determined by the waxing and waning of the moon, and then the mourning rites that had to be gone through, as though it were all a matter of course" (176).

Here we have not only the interruption but the inversion of the protocols of an adequate historicization, for death, putatively the end of life, precedes the life of which it would be the end. What

is being mourned here in the household's *butsudan* (which here figures as a Buddhist shrine in the innermost recesses of the domus)
is not a past but a future, and that not merely in the mode of a certain prolepsis. These corpses—in the case of the Egyptian, for example, sheer exteriority—are what is most interior to Tomiko's
"woman"; her children, the guarantee of her historicization, are
not merely dead on arrival, but "before" any possibility of arrival,
always already dead meat, history. Death, the end of life, precedes
life; the sheer material exteriority of the corpse is what is most interior. No wonder, then, that Aki's reaction is precisely the exteri-
orization of interiority: "On the way back from Tomiko's house . . .
Aki vomited twice" (176). What then of the domesticity and interiority of the figure of the woman (*oku*, which in Japanese designates woman, as "the Mrs.," quite explicitly as the very interiority of
domesticity)? Tomiko convinces herself that the regularity of the
regulative nomos can be restored and sustained through an accomplished mourning, which would be at the same time a successful,
accomplished parturition. For Aki, however, it is around the figure
of the woman that the Law of binary opposition is *essentially* destabilized. And the binary is destabilized precisely in the confusion or
coincidence of parturition and death: "The blistering cries of things
that leave the womb and the gossamer-weak whimpers from the
beds in the old people's home must melt and run together somewhere in the sky at night" (178). So is the traumatic nightmare
(177), which involves the essentially transgression of boundaries, a
nightmare of parturition or of death?

    If Aki's relation to Tomiko revolves around an impossible his-
toricization, a relation to death before life, her relation to the dying
Setsuko is structured as a premature, proleptic mourning. Dying of
a cancer perhaps induced by radiation, Setsuko has been hospitalized
before the cultural accomplishment of a certain domesticity, before
the consummation of marriage. Her husband, like every Father present only by virtue of his absence on the cultural work of the world
(195–96), sends her postcards of the Sphinx. Setsuko herself is the
object of a proleptic mourning: "Her meagre flesh hung around
her bones as if it were some sort of thick wrapping paper covering

her temporarily. What I saw that day deep inside her were the thin burned-up bones; what I heard was the brittle crumbling of their white calcinated remains" (179). We shall see a very nearly identical description of hibakusha with radiation sickness in Ōta Yōko; it is probably entirely unnecessary to note a correspondence to the image of the person with AIDS as it has been figured in innumerable representations. As in Ōta, as in the cases of people in the terminal stages of AIDS, what is at issue in the relation between Aki and Setsuko is the relation of a nonrelation, or of the impossibility of relation, the relation to the corpse. No surprise, then, that Setsuko, unlike Tomiko, does not speak.

The corpse, that scrap of the Real around which the historicization of every mourning is structured, can only figure for thought as that essentially unthinkable excess or surplus that is materiality in its absolute nontranscendence. First, no intersubjective relation with the corpse is thinkable or even imaginable; second, the corpse necessarily figures as what exceeds the integral unity of the Imaginary "body," precisely because the corpse is the "is what it is" of what is. The corpse is therefore the surplus or excess of identity, and indeed, of being; in its materiality, the surplus of ideality. At once, the corpse is both the occasion for, and the necessity of, historicization, as well as the impossibility of any historicization adequate to its object. The corpse is an absolute resistance to transcendence, the Real that is unsublatable. Insofar as it is a "figure" or "image," the corpse is the figure or image of the impossibility of figurality. But the corpse is also that without which there can be no work of mourning, no thought of the binary opposition of life and death. The corpse, in itself singular and therefore that scrap which refuses predication and judgment absolutely, is nevertheless that which is the impossible condition of possibility for every idealization, every historicization. This impossible relation, this impossibility of relation, or this relation of nonrelation, or this radical alterity, of the corpse is thus the ground of every work of mourning, every historicization, every work of culture.

For Aki, this relation of nonrelation to the corpse is impossible. "The Rite" is punctuated by a series of traumatic memories, untranscendable as trauma, each of which is introduced by a repetition (which echoes one of the constant thematics in the so-called "atomic bomb literature"):

> Aki has never seen Junko's dead body. . . .
> Aki has never seen Kazue's dead body.
> Nor Emiko's dead body.
> No, nor Ikuko's.
> Nor has she ever come across anyone else who witnessed their end or verified the deaths of Junko or Kiyoko or Kazue or Yayoi. . . .
> In the devastated school ground a mound of black earth had been raised and on top of it was just one plain wooden marker. Buried beneath in unglazed urns, indiscriminately gathered up with all those other deaths, must I recognize the deaths of Junko and Kiyoko and Kazue as well? Even so, if the dead, as they say, are never truly dead and will not rest in peace until the appropriate rites of mourning are performed for them, then the deaths of Junko and of Kiyoko and Kazue are not yet, so to speak, fully accomplished. (181–84)

There is an apparently double problematic at work here. First, there is the problematic of a certain "empiricism" (although not of those forms of empiricism that, in their appeals to the immanent legibility of experience, deny that they have a problematic at all). Here it is a question of witnessing and verification; as in the case of the Faurisson controversy (and thereby of the entire *Historikerstreit*), what is necessarily impossible is any empirical verification of the existence of the object itself. In the disappearance of the object, in the disappearance that *is* the "object" of historiographical discourse, the very possibility for witnessing and verification disappears with and as that "object." Such "objects" become the black holes of the historical Imaginary, the very nihility of their objectness, in annihilating the very possibility of empirical experience, overtakes and obliterates that very objectness.[40] Thus, any witness here can be only a witness to the very impossibility of testimony, verification becomes the verification of the very impossibility of verification. What is absent from the historiographical Imaginary, and invisible before the epistemological Gaze of the historian, is the scrap of the Real (here the corpse) that would putatively convince one of the existence of the Real itself. What is in question, therefore, is neither a relation, a relation of nonrelation, nor in fact any possibility for relation at all, but the utter irrelevance of relationality altogether. We are presented with an utter outside-of-rationality or the logos, an unthinkable madness, insofar as it must be thought of as an outside with no relation whatsoever to an inside.

Concomitantly, we are presented with the problematic of the radical contingency, the absolute nondiscrimination of historicity and materiality, of the singularity of the proper name, which can never be reduced to the sign of an autonomous ego, individual, or subject. "Junko," "Kazue," "Emiko," "Ikuko," "Kiyoko": these proper nouns in the propriety of their naming, become what Lyotard has called "anonyms." It is as anonyms alone that they mark a singularity that can never be reduced to the assumption of a universal individuality or subjectivity; these anonymic names are not particularities that belong to the universal, which would amount to a humanism of the dead. Rather, these anonyms mark that singularity which is the site of the impossibility of predication, the site at which predication is exhausted in an infinite congestion of the proper. To this exhaustion of the infinite singularity and difference of an unverifiable empirical that is beyond all testimony save the testimony of the anonym itself, I think I am following Maurice Blanchot in assigning the term "destitution."[41]

Necessarily, and tautologically, this destitution of the empirical, which makes the project of an accomplished work of mourning impossible, is the effect and actualization of a certain existentiality, an existentiality marked as 6 August 1945, the event—advent—of the Outside "as such"; "that time" (*ano toki; tōji*). Sunset on "a quiet peaceful Saturday," a "fitting end to a fine summer's day," will find an asymmetrical analogue in Aki's memory "of that other summer's day," when "the bright evening glow was not caused simply by the setting sun" (186). But the event around which this text, and so many other texts, including the textuality of our lives ever after forever, is structured, is a *missed* reality (to which, as Lacan says, the

traumatic neurosis—an unaccomplished historicization—is homage):
"The morning, the great flash, the big bang, the squall of wind, the
fire . . . all these I can remember very clearly, but what happened
to me next? That was a blank in her memory that Aki was not able
to fill in" (186). The event, in itself and as such, cannot be historicized because it cannot be narrated or remembered. It is precisely in
this syncope in the historiographical operation that the intuition of
the Kantian a priori, within which alone objects can be constituted
for historical knowing, becomes radically impossible: *what is left is the
intuition of the aporia of the a priori.* It is for this reason that "if I could
catch the real nature of that thing and fling the fullness of my anger
and hate at it, I would not be in torment to this day, well over ten
years after, tied to this fierce anger that still finds no proper outlet. I
would not be tortured by this nameless hate that yet finds no clear
object" (194–95). The impossibility of constituting and verifying
the event as an object for knowing lays waste to an entire series (a
narrative really) of perception, objectification, predication, judgment, understanding, and, finally, the Bildung of the historiographical operation. What becomes singularly impossible is the
achievement of identity in the *speculum* of a history construed according to its effects as the artifacts of material culture:

> Even if it has only a tin roof I don't mind! I want to sleep somewhere
> that isn't out on the bare ground!
>   I don't mind if it isn't in a glass! I want some clean water that
> you're not afraid to drink!
>   Even a piece so small it fits into the hollow of my hand, I don't
> mind! I want to see myself in something you could call a mirror! (194)

The witness to the event, the witness to the impossibility of witnessing, becomes the vampire, the ghost, the undead deprived of
all specularity, of Imaginary identity. Here, ultimately, the "self,"
too, becomes an aporia, the aporetic autoaffectivity that is the aporia of every empiricism, an aporia resistant to every intuition:

> Aki began to suspect uneasily that the hazy something that had lost its
> clean outlines might be her own self. . . .
>   . . . The rite that should have been performed and never was,

and my unassuaged thirst for it, I must recognize as the beginning of a questioning of "being" that I must now develop. Wherein lies the realness of things? Can you say that a thing that's really there and that you can be sure of is one your eyes can see, your hands can touch, your skin can feel? The things in your consciousness, that you can neither see nor touch, are they less truly there?

But what degree of realness is there in things your eyes can see, your hands can touch, or your skin can feel? (195)

These thematics all intersect in the image of the disintegration, ultimately the utter annihilation, of the domestic comforts of the domus. At once *Heimat, habitus, ie, uchi,* and "home," the domus is the Imaginary site toward which is directed the nostalgia of what Lyotard calls "*homo re-domesticus*," the site of a rhythmicity or abiding (*tsune*) that would be sufficient prophylaxis against the depredations of historicity.[42] This nostalgia for the domus is a nostalgia for a lost ontological plentitude (or the plentitude we once called ontology), a virtual *jouissance.* But it is a nostalgia for that which never was: the domus exists only in the wake of its disintegration and annihilation, the domus is only ever a lost site of identity. Thus Aki seeks "a proper place for me to go back to," but of which she asks, "What exactly in that place would I be going home to? If there is something there that's fitting to return to, I want it to be something that endures unchanged and transcends time. Something of which it may be said, now *that* at least is certain. People should return to something that, no matter what may happen, will endure and still be seen as the true root and source of what they are" (191). Undoubtedly entire discursive formations, on place, identity, women, maternity, the abiding folk and culture, intersect in Aki's nostalgic reflection on a domus defined essentially by its imperturbable resistance to historicity. Thus, the security of the domus is really the possibility for any security whatsoever; the security of the domus, Takenishi's text discloses, is the possibility for security as such.

So it is not merely that the event can be encoded as an unhappy accident that has befallen the domus, which homo re-domesticus in an act of will might restore to its primal purity, the resurrection of an original integrity that would be the primordial site of cultural ground itself. Rather, what has befallen the domus is the contingency, the absolute insecurity, of historicity *itself*; what has befallen the domus is *apocalyptic* contingency. Aki herself entertains the possibility of restoring the domus to its primordial and eternal security. Gazing "on the vast multitude of dead in all the chaos of that ruined ground, laid waste and desolate by someone or by something yet unknown," she speculates that perhaps "it is only a temporary phenomenon! I kept on pursuing the original appearance of that place as it had been before, and as I was sure it would be again" (192). Perhaps the apocalyptic event can be transcended. But, no, she realizes, the apocalypse is forever, and whenever. Hereafter, Hiroshima will be haunted by a past that is also a future. Beyond the untenable consolations of daily life in postwar Hiroshima, there will be the unfigurable figure of destitution (193–94).

We must go further here. The place of the domus becomes the nonplace, the site, of destitution itself. Henceforth, it is not merely that the radical contingency of historicity is occluded by the consolations of the daily life of place and domus (although indeed it is), but that the domus is *at the same time* the site of destitution:

> That place of mine that was so beautiful—if it was truly mine, then that same place when hideously changed by someone or some force unknown to me was surely also mine. To the question of which is really the true place, I cannot answer now with any confidence. If one speaks in terms of a phenomenon, then both were that. If asked which was reality, I am inclined to say that both were also that. But surely what I called unchanging, the abiding source one can always go home to, must be something richer far than either, rejecting neither of them but transcending both. It must be something solidly sustained by an imperturbable order, although it may reveal itself under the varying aspects of separate phenomena. Yes, I shall no doubt go to that place again, but I will not be going home. . . . To my regret, that imperturbable order is now known to me only within the world of wishful intimations. But I must know if it really exists. If I could know it, even in a flash of intuition, then perhaps I would no longer be the prey of this eery stillness that takes hold of me. I would be freed then from my terror of being sucked into the void that blocks

out the light and of falling down, down, down into that black abyss. I want to know. (199–200)

Here, place, as the imperturbable order that would be the ground of a desire to know, which in Takenishi is undoubtedly something more than a mere epistemophilia, becomes the very impossibility of an "imperturbable order," of order as such. The ground, this ruined ground, will henceforth be the apocalypse itself.

Four Itineraries in Search of a Narrative

Ōta Yōko's *City of Corpses* traces a congeries of trajectories or itineraries in search of a narrative, which is to say in search of the sense and meaning narrative promises. The terms "trajectories" and "itineraries" here indicate both, and *at once*, that attempt and the irremediable failure of that attempt. In the first instance, these trajectories and itineraries in search of a narrative are therefore concerned with the putative essential possibility for historiography, with the possibility for the historiographical altogether, for the successive possibilities of testimony, witnessing, making sense, the possibilities of historicizing and domesticating the event (as such), that would be the sole ground of historical consciousness. These itineraries mark both the *necessity* and the necessarily concomitant *impossibility* of that attempt. Within this general consideration of the essential possibility for the historiographical altogether, there are four analogous itineraries I want to retrace. It is, of course, extremely schematic to isolate four itineraries here; furthermore, although they are never reducible to the same, they intersect and coincide at critical junctures. Their separation, as I represent them here, is quite obviously fictive.

First, there is an itinerary of the phenomenological or of a putative personal experience and its testimony. But here the phenomenological, or experience, is a passage to its own innermost limit. It is not merely a matter of refusing the phenomenological or the personal and embracing an objectivity (however construed), but of the experience of the limit as the limit of experience, the experience of a limit (which is not some generalized "horizon" out there somewhere) at which the construction of experience as the validation of a subjectivist autonomy is surpassed, or—in a very specific sense— "transcended." What is at stake in Ōta, as in Takenishi, is the impossibility of the intuition of the a priori, the intuition of the aporia. This phenomenological passage is not a passage *to* any alterity whatever (such as a state of being, grace, meaning, or truth), but a passage that is itself historicity and sociality, what Christopher Fynsk designates as "finite transcendence," the passage "through" a materiality that can only be figured as the surplus of meaning, interpretation, and comprehensibility.[43]

Second, I shall try to retrace the itinerary or trajectory of a secession or retreat from the stark horrors of destitution in search of the redemptions of the Imaginary domus, the primordial ground of culture, of technē, of every domestic economy. This primordial ground of culture has classically been conceived, at least in what counts as "modernity," as a separation from nature, which is at the same time a rooting of culture in "nature" (because it is a matter of a *relation*—whether of continuity, discontinuity, or opposition—between culture and nature). Ostensibly, then, there is here a nostalgia for an Imaginary prehistory. What is in question in Ōta is the possibility of a "culture" that is not a separation from anything, but an originary separation, a primordial disjunction, that gives the lie to any nostalgia for the domesticity of the cultural domus. It is a matter of technē, of the conjunction of use with need. Thus "culture" is revealed to be the fact of nonrelationality *itself*, of historicity. In Ōta, this secession is encoded as a relation to the historical Imaginary, or what she calls "Japan."

Third, I therefore read *City of Corpses* to project the itinerary of a questioning concerning the possibility of a geopolitical—institutional, scientific social—historiography adequate not only to the narration but to the narrativization and comprehensibility of the event of 6 August 1945. Concomitantly, there is in Ōta a thought of nuclear terror as the ground of the political. At stake is the question of the possibility of any teratology adequate to the incommensurability of what it purports to represent, and thereby to give meaning to and thus transcend the apocalyptic destitution of the historico-social. This itinerary is at once a necessary but also a necessarily impossible peregrination. These first three itineraries effectively define what I have called destitution as the insistence of the existential, as materiality, that is to say.

Fourth, Ōta's text describes, and is, the trajectory of a writing, the trajectory of the writing it in fact is. Here, the writing of *City of Corpses*, quite explicitly thematized in and as *City of Corpses*, is bound to the various thematics of witnessing and testimony, as well as to their necessary impossibility (where one can only testify to the impossibility of testimony, witness to the impossibility of witnessing); to the appropriation of witness and testimony in an attempt to occlude that to which witness witnesses and testimony testifies; to the thematics of art and transcendence (including a nostalgia for landscape and the literary, nostalgia for a literary "nature"). In *City of Corpses*, writing—and the writing of *City of Corpses*—is not merely a "response" to the force of the existential and of existentiality as such (in which aspect, the writing is a correspondence of representation to its objects and therefore a relation, however problematic); "writing" here is also *essential* to the intuition of the aporia, writing is the passage "to" the impossibility of thought and representation. Here writing becomes itself the limit-experience. This writing would therefore be what Blanchot calls "research," a relation of nonrelation, a historiography that not only "acknowledges" its own historicity (still assuming the ideal adequacy of the concept to the thinking of what must be thought), but a *thought of* the impossibility of an adequate conceptuality for the historical.[44]

The Phenomenological Itinerary

When it is a question of the aporetic limit of the phenomenological—which is to say, the necessarily phenomenological experi-

ence of the limit, or impossibility, of phenomenological experience
—then it is first of all a question of temporality. It is a question of an
essential disturbance of the intuition of the transcendental a priori.
That this disturbance, interruption, syncope, or discontinuity is "essential" means that it interrupts or disturbs forevermore the commonsense intuition of time as extension or continuity traversing
past, present, and future, a commonsense intuition that is constitutive of any (transcendental) *sensus communis*. What demands to be
thought here is the difference, the singularity, the radical discontinuity, the nontranscendence that is the impossible but necessary
ground of temporality construed as extension or continuity. This
interruption or discontinuity can only be thought of *as* the interruption or discontinuity of a continuity, in relation to continuity:
the insistence or exigency of the existential can only be thought as
an *essentially* aporetic insistence.[45] In other words, what needs to be
thought is the intuition of the aporia of the intuition of the a priori.

In *City of Corpses*, this limit is thought as the punctuality of the
event: Hiroshima, 8:15:17 A.M., 6 August 1945. This in turn is
thought as the *conjunction* of a geopolitical, "macrotemporal," even
"world-historical," discursive construction of temporality *with* the
"microtemporal" construction of (a)temporality in the abiding
rhythmicity of daily life: the apocalypse begins at home. But this
unique, singular event, in its punctuality and absolute difference, is
also thought as an infinite punctuality, as an indifferent "whenever."
This infinite punctuality of the indifferent "whenever" is figured
both as the permanent present possibility of nuclear holocaust (it
can always happen again—whenever), and as radiation sickness in
its absolute contingency for the hibakusha and their genetic descendants. *City of Corpses* demands a thinking of all these temporalities *together*, as the disjunct simultaneity of difference and indifference, of the punctuality of the here and now with the infinite
punctuality of the indiscriminate whenever.

The temporalities of 6 August 1945 are registered in *City of
Corpses* as phenomenological affects that cannot be reduced to
merely psychological categories. (Perhaps they could be thought as
the psychological or subjective *inscriptions* of a logic.) Consider the

temporality of these affects, drawn, of course, from Freud's *Beyond the Pleasure Principle*, and presented as a very reductive schematism: they are of only provisional use here. Fear (*Furcht*) demands an object, something to be afraid of; fright (*Schreck*) takes one by surprise; anxiety (*Angst*) is "a particular state of expecting the danger or preparing for it, even though it may be an unknown one."[46] Fear is entirely caught up in the anticipation of a future; fright, as surprise, is bound to the happening or *Geschehen* of the event in the here and now; anxiety, that fabled affect once held to be characteristic of "our" time, implies the time of an infinite punctuality. Both anticipation and surprise, anxiety demands an infinite attention to the destitution of what is, the thought of the apocalypse now, forever, whenever. Fear is the inscription of a continuity with regard to which, however disastrous it may be, one might still imagine a teratology adequate to the object; fright marks a radical discontinuity, the eruption of the Real in the Imaginary, an absolute and irremediable rupture; anxiety inscribes an impossible continuity, as Nishida would have it, the continuity of discontinuity (*hirenzoku no renzoku*), the illimitable, persistent, and unavoidable insistence of the existential, the "time of the Real" or of materiality as the absolute contingency of what is, the guarantee of a historicity that can never be recapitulated in any continuity except as its aporetic limit. The time of anxiety is the time of metamorphosis.

Now certainly, before 6 August 1945 in Hiroshima, and before 9 August 1945 in Nagasaki, there was something to be afraid of. In spite of various conjectures that Hiroshima might be spared the horror visited upon other Japanese cities, the very fact that Hiroshima and Nagasaki were among the few cities *not* firebombed guaranteed the fear of extensive firebombing. Indeed, residents of Hiroshima had spent the better part of the previous night in air-raid shelters; the all-clear had sounded less than an hour before the blast. One of the constant themes produced by the hibakusha in Hiroshima and Nagasaki is this anticipation, this sense of a predictable fate (for Ōta's account, see 166–67, 182). But in the event, of course, the event was entirely surprising, frightening. Nothing had equipped the residents of Hiroshima or Nagasaki to be prepared for, to explain or make sense of the event; it was, *absolutely*, an *anomaly*:

> How could everything in our vicinity have been so transformed in one instant? We hadn't the slightest idea. Perhaps it hadn't been an air raid. In my daze, I had a different idea: that it might have no connection with the war, that it might be something that occurs at the end of the world, when the globe disintegrates. As children, we had read about such things in books. (185)

Such a thought bespeaks the utter impossibility of comprehending the event *except as cosmic apocalypse*, itself necessarily beyond comprehensibility. Indeed, even the war itself would be encoded in "childish nonsense," a reflection recollected in the memory of the bombing, in the wake of the event:

> And this huge war itself—perhaps it wasn't something that some human beings had started against other human beings? Otherwise it was too tragic, too horrifying. Perhaps it wasn't war at all, but the latest cosmic phenomenon? So many months and years had passed since the world began; perhaps the globe wasn't able any longer to rein in all its emotions and had handed the reins over to the world of natural phenomena? There is even, it seems, a term "universal gravitation"; this war must have arisen out of that supernatural force. It is neither a war of aggression nor, as Japan often said, a war for control of the world, nor a war simply for the sake of East Asia. It may not be a passing vanity of that sort; instead, it may be a philosophical, a cosmic phantasm that has taken the form of war and is on the prowl. With truly fearsome power, with truly fearsome sadism. Unless that were the case, an event of this magnitude probably would never have taken place. The fate of the cosmos itself, no doubt, is to burn out and then become colder than ice; then again blaze, be destroyed, collapse; then wander anew; then shed silent tears of sadness and anger. The process of the earth's self-destruction, so to speak, might have taken the form of war. (211)

The immediate reaction to the instantaneous and absolute transformation of what is into an illimitable destitution is one of an infinite fright that strips the subject of its every affect; what is there to be afraid of at the end of the world? "Where we were, things were

quiet, hushed. (The newspaper wrote that there was 'instant pan-
demonium,' but that was a preconceived notion on the part of the
writer. In fact, an eerie stillness settled, so still that one wondered
whether people, trees, and plants hadn't all died at one fell swoop.)"
(185). Later in the day, destitution becomes, or takes the place of,
the "ontological condition":

> We could not conceive of the day's events as being related in any way
> to the war. We had been flattened by a force—arbitrary and violent—
> that wasn't war. Moreover, fellow countrymen did not particularly
> encourage one another, nor did they console one another. They be-
> haved submissively and said not a word. No one showed up to tend
> the injured; no one came to tell us how or where to pass the night.
> We were simply on our own. (192; see also 189, 202)

In other words, what is implied in this destitution is that the
affect of fright (the impossibility of registering the happening of the
event according to the transcendental a priori) is both the very limit
of a temporal comprehensibility *and* (thereby and vice versa) the
aporetic limit of affectivity altogether: "We were not afraid of the
atomic bomb. We had no time to think about being afraid. And
even afterward we were not afraid. We probably won't be afraid until two or three years have passed" (253). The time of destitution is
the infinite punctuality of the whenever of a radical contingency.
For the event remains a permanent possibility: in the countryside
to which Ōta has retreated in the days after the bombing, an air-
raid siren sounds, recalling the permanent possibility of an attack
(262), and thereby of nuclear annihilation. The time of fright, as it
were, opens upon the time of anxiety.

The radical contingency of the whenever of an infinite punctuality makes a nonsense of every phenomenological apprehension.
It is not merely that "in order to escape being injured by the atomic
bomb, nothing was of any use except not being in Hiroshima"
(213), but also that the most immediate effects (cuts and burns) de-
pended entirely upon chance, giving rise to a desperate but impossible attempt to "speculate the elements," to establish an explana-
tory causality, to explain the inexplicable. Thus, death comes inexplicably to those who have not been burned, or have been only

slightly burned, or whose cuts were horizontal rather than vertical; most generally, it is "the phenomenon of completely unanticipated death," a death the restorations of no narrative can explain (244–50). This puts paid to every notion of death as the consummation of life. Moreover, this radical contingency remains a permanent possibility for the hibakusha in yet another respect, as the death in life, the death that is life, of "atomic-bomb sickness,"—which means that the event is not merely punctual but extensive. In this sense, the bombing never stops; and all of this is inexplicably new to the hibakusha. This death-that-is-life of radiation sickness is constituted as a syndrome, its symptoms (fever, loss of energy, apathy, loss of hair, loss of blood, tonsillitis, diarrhea) in their appearance or advent defying a phenomenology of temporal causality (such as what is called medical science). Both as "unanticipated death," and in the contingencies of the symptomological syndrome, radiation sickness is experienced according to the same phenomenological aporiae as is AIDS, as an unavoidable but ultimately unspecifiable insistence of existentiality: "The damage caused by the atomic bomb is peculiar in these ways: people do not feel pain immediately in their bodies, and the symptoms do not manifest themselves for a long while" (159). The status of the HIV seropositive and the hibakusha, in respect of a certain anxiety—the radical contingency of a punctuality of infinite extension—is the same.

What this amounts to, registered in and as the material existence of the hibakusha or HIV seropositive, is the intuition of the temporal aporia of the event in its uncontainable, unbounded extension. And it is this that makes the historicization of the work of mourning impossible, for both "past" and "future" become essentially indissociable from an apocalyptic present (which is, as such, of course essentially ungraspable, essentially absent). Here, then, is a temporal destitution, the indifferent ground of the whenever.

This "phenomenological" intuition of the temporal aporia, of the indifferent ground of every difference (or therefore of pure difference), is at once the ground and limit of historical consciousness *and* the ground and limit of autoaffectivity and what is called subjectivity.

There were dead bodies wherever we went. Dead bodies virtually blocked the road we were walking on, though it was not really a road. Almost all of the bodies had burns, so even alive they had given off a foul odor. Half-decayed, the dead bodies sent wafting in the air an acid smell, as of a crematorium. Some of the dead bodies seemed to have only just died, and the salve that had been used to treat their burns gleamed wet and white in the sunlight. Unmoved, unafraid, we walked amid the corpses. . . .

By then I was accustomed to dead bodies. Everyone was. Even on the sixth itself, the day the bomb fell, people did not feel any great pain from their own severe injuries, and there was virtually no anguish in our hearts. The dead bodies themselves did not show agony —neither the beautiful bodies of children that looked alive nor the bodies that had begun to decompose. Nor did the people passing by revive our anguish. We didn't think of connecting this situation in any way with the war. It was as if we had lost even the ability to think. (225–26)

In the event, Hiroshima became instantaneously a thanatopolis, a "tangle" of corpses so dense that when the narrator's sister and mother project an escape to the nearby island of Nojima (rumored to be a repository for corpses from Hiroshima) via Ujina or Honkawa, the narrator is skeptical of the project, for "even supposing Sister and Mother got as far as Ujina or Honkawa, there was no telling how many corpses they would have to trample on, street after street, before they got that far" (214); the very geography of hell is mapped in corpses. In other words, corpses are all there is, an infinite congestion of the totality; there is in Hiroshima no outside of abjection. But if there is no "outside" of abjection in the narrator's Hiroshima (and we have seen, and shall see again, the death-that-is-life of the hibakusha differs in no essential respect from the abjection of the corpse), if all that is *is* abjection, then the corpse can only be a pure surplus or excess. The purity of this surplus cannot, however, be construed as a simple negativity; rather, it must be thought as the excess of every binary. To return to one of the themes of the discussion of Takenishi's "The Rite," we must recognize that the corpse does not refer back ("historically") to the life that once animated it, nor is it *merely* the trace of an absent presence; rather than being the remains of a subjectivity, the corpse is essentially anonymous, rendering vain every work of mourning. The corpse is not, that is to say, the figure of ideality, the domestication of the soul. It is a pure image, the pure possibility of image, not the image *of* anything.[47] The "corpse" therefore pertains to our historicity as something essentially other than the memento mori of the work of mourning, other than what befalls a subject, which would render the corpse the object of, or at least occasion for, an affectivity. "Unmoved, unafraid, we walked amid the corpses." Here the corpse, which is not merely irreducible to signification or to meaning or to sense, but *is* that very irreducibility, is neither merely the image of an irremediable destitution, but that destitution in its essential nontranscendence: which is beyond every affect. The corpse is the utter vacancy of the ontological, the vacancy that takes the place of every possible ontology.

Let us be obvious and note further that the corpse is not merely that which is deprived of all instrumentality, but is the essential impossibility of any instrumental relation, of instrumental relationally altogether, first of all as the impossibility of that instrumental relation called intersubjectivity. It is the surplus of use, need, and their coincidence in Brauch. The corpse is thus the surplus of the cultural as such, the outside of the quotidian; but it is not thereby returned to "nature" in any mysticism. If the corpse figures as the outside of culture, it is not thereby merely an alternative term in a binary (for it is of the corpse's recuperation within that binary that the work of mourning is meant to convince us). The corpse, in its noninstrumentality, therefore figures as the "outside" of culture and technē, as the "outside" of the logos, of the possibility for rationality altogether, as *madness*, as an essential disturbance in the possibility for making sense of things.

The corpses of Hiroshima and Nagasaki, in their infinite anonymous and noninstrumental singularity, therefore figure as pure difference, by which I mean a difference that can be recuperated in no binary, in no dialectic. Strictly speaking, this pure difference is unthinkable: it is a question of the singularity of what Nishida called the "individual thing" (*kobutsu*), which in its materiality must be thought as the exhaustion of predication in the infinite congestion of the proper. Pure difference, and that pure difference which is the corpse, must be thought as a separation, but not a separation-from; it is therefore an originary separation. It is not prepredicative in the sense of an original presentation, but—if anything—postpredicative or apredicative, the surplus of predication and sense. In its material, existential objectivity, it is the surplus of any possibility of objectification. Insofar as it is an object (a "corpse"), it is an object that is the image of the impossibility of objectification. This unremitting pure difference of the "tangle" of corpses that Hiroshima *is* in *City of Corpses* is an *indifference* beyond any possibility of affectivity, as Ōta records over and over again (and therefore, again, an absolute resistance to the possibility of mourning or historicization). But this pure difference is also indifferent in the sense of an unrelieved quiescence, of being without agency. Corpses are indifferent in the sense as well of being *indiscriminate*, the figures of a radical contingency: "The young man was dead. His was the first corpse I had seen that hadn't bled at all and that had no burns" (225). Thus, too, with radiation sickness, death comes indiscriminately, in a kind of apocalyptic promiscuity, an indiscriminate discrimination. Now, for the indifference of the pure difference of the city of corpses—which occupies the site of what once we knew as ontology—there is a term, of course: "entropy," the indifferent ground of pure difference, of an originary separation (what Nishida called *mu no basho* or *rekishiteki kūkan*).[48] In this sense, "destitution" designates the indifference of pure difference.

Therefore, the corpse, the image (object) of its very unobjectifiability, in the indifference of its pure difference, reveals the absolute and unbearable destitution of entropy to be a pure historicity (sometimes encoded as absolute loss, which can be misleading in that it suggests the mourning of subjects who have lost something). The entropy of this pure historicity, in its destitution, is at once (and here the simultaneity of the conjunction is essential), the ground *of* historical consciousness and the unthinkable, unbearable limit *of* historical consciousness. It is literally unbearable in the sense of being the experience of the impossibility of experience, an absolutely impersonal "personal experience": the *epochē*.

And here is the disturbing thought: this entropy, this destitution, this pure historicity, this infinite punctuality of the indifference of pure difference, is thereby, and originarily, a pure sociality, the ground of the social as such. What is revealed in the *City of Corpses* is that the death of the other (a pure or absolute nonrelation or nonrelationality altogether) is the ground of the social: an unbearable thought, as Blanchot noted in his reading of Bataille that I have quoted. The relation to the corpse is the relation to the absolutely Other—a pure nonrelationality, therefore, uncorrupted by any version of intersubjectivity, untranscendable in any thought of community or sensus communis. In other words, any possibility for sociality stands upon the untenable ground of its impossibility. The destitution of this pure sociality is unbearable, both because it is strictly speaking unthinkable (as simultaneous condition of both possibility and limit for sociality), but also (or perhaps it comes to the same thing) as that which a certain "we" *are*, the abjects of community. This destitution, this abjection that is the ground of sociality, is registered in *City of Corpses* as the aporia—the impossibility—of affectivity, or, yet more strongly, as the loss of desire, aphanisis. This impossibility of affectivity and this aphanisis, this abjection, all figure as the absolute ground of every attempt to reconstitute sociality among the hibakusha. This is a recurrent—psychoanalysis would say obsessive—theme of *City of Corpses*.

The destitution of the bombings extends to the entirety of the war itself: "Sadly, the war had left everyone dazed and exhausted. As the end of the war approached and even before the atomic bombs, Japan itself had already fallen to the mental state epitomized by expressionless faces" (169). Thus, "the exhaustion of a dazed populace made for more deaths that day in Hiroshima; it piled up the corpses" (165). In the event, and in fleeing the house, the narrator leaves behind the goods to which she was attached, for "like a person beyond such desires I did not reach for them. It would be better to say that I had lost interest in the belongings than that I had given up on them. . . . This hollowness, almost numbness, lasted a long while" (186). Repeatedly, and frequently parenthetically, the text is punctuated by this reminder or this glimpse of the absence of an affectivity: "Victims of the atomic bomb have vacant expressions" (e.g., 217). Or: "[N]o matter how strange you looked, people did not laugh. Nor did they show sympathy. For no matter how sad the shape you were in, people no longer felt they had to show sympathy" (225). "Living corpses" (273), and the phrase is something rather more than a metaphor, the hibakusha become something other than human: "The axe of fate . . . fell, with no warning, on all our heads alike; so it would have been fitting had death, too, come to all alike. Perhaps those who survived were some kind of insect, were not human" (252). Indeed, it is this very lack of affectivity that becomes the index of the corpse that the hibakusha already is, both *Doppelgänger* and identity:

> One of the symptoms of atomic bomb disease is an expressionless face. It is not, I think, something that develops after one contracts radiation sickness; it has been in evidence ever since August 6. It is the expressionless face of imbecility, the face of the idiot. The expressionless face of the imbecile has become a state of mind, and it is this very condition that manifests itself in the victims of this calamity, setting them apart. . . .
>
> But the shadow of death crossed before our very eyes, returned, passed on. Alongside one's live self stood one's dead self. There are no words to describe it. (253)

Or: "I looked about me dazedly, half expecting to see my dead body stretched out somewhere" (182). Thus, "Now subject, now object, we victims could not help feeling that death was forever tugging at us" (177).

In a disjunct simultaneity, the hibakusha in an essential abjection is neither alive nor dead, neither present nor absent, neither inside nor outside the human, but the surplus of every binary. Both social and the impossibility of sociality, neither social nor the impossibility of the social, the hibakusha—as the corpse but as also something other than a corpse, as pure surplus but also as the surplus of that material surplus—is the very transgression of transcendence, of destitution: inhabiting an impossible, unbearable site, the hibakusha is the incarnation of the relation of nonrelation. Both. Neither. Both both and neither. Neither both nor neither. Here, then, the social can have no ground, least of all the ground of affectivity as such, save the very impossibility of ground. In their historicity, *as* their historicity, the hibakusha are situated otherwise than as the objects of an appropriate mourning.

Yet the hibakusha nevertheless become, in their abjection, the objects for a proleptic, albeit impossible mourning. They become first of all, as objects of the bombing, the objects for a magisterial Gaze, in the first instance for the American camera; a certain scientific, medical, anthropological, historiographical Gaze. The B-29s return, but now as tourists (191, 202). As epistemological tourists, to be sure, who like all tourists are in search of an object for the gaze. But this epistemophiliac tourism, this objectification, in its very sympathy and humanitarianism, establishes, or *re*establishes, the difference between the community of the living and the abject objects of a proleptic mourning. It is precisely in turning the epistemophiliac gaze upon the hibakusha that the ruined ground of the historico-social is *occluded*; the victim, qua object, qua image, veils the unbearable ground of historicity and sociality precisely by "re"-instituting the binary:

> What was strange was the relationship that arose between victims and nonvictims. From the first, the average person treated the injured, from whom he differed only in not being injured, almost as if they had always been dirty beggars. He was arrogant in words and attitude and treated them as inferiors. I could not help being struck both by this psychology and also by the psychology whereby victims as victims became absolutely servile, as if they had always been pathetic creatures, even though only two or three days had passed since they had been burned out of house and home. (217)

At the end of an extended discussion of "refugee mentality" (231–34), the narrator notices that clerks selling bus tickets some days later "simply did not respond to refugees who wished to inquire about various things. The refugees stood alone" (234–35). And this status, or this impossibility of having a status, has its institutional sanction, for "we couldn't go anywhere without papers certifying that we were victims" (208). What is in question in the abjectification of the victim or the refugee is the production of a social surplus, a work by which a community of the clean and healthy is confirmed in its putative identity. Whether we are speaking of the hibakusha and their genetic descendants, or of people living with AIDS, it is important to note that we are speaking of two victimizations. The first is the material violence brought to bear on bodies, either the immediate and long-term physical effects of the bombings or the opportunistic infections that are an effect of the suppression of the immune system by HIV. The second victimization is the discursive constitution of the "victim" as the abject object of a proleptic work of mourning. It is precisely the exile of this second victimization that has been refused ever since the enunciation of the Denver Principles in 1983 by people *living* with AIDS.

And—equally precisely—it is this refusal of victimization that gives the lie to that logic of integration which is the ideological ground of liberal humanism and, indeed, humanitarianism. For liberal humanism projects an Imaginary totality—the human community—within which the abject is reintegrated *only on condition that the abjection is accepted or in fact affirmed*. This is precisely the logic of integration that we saw in Nishida's address to the National Policy Research Association: you are accepted into the community of the "we" only insofar as you confirm your abject otherness, only insofar as you accept your essentially passive objectivity. Which is no integration at all, of course. Thus, in the cases both of Hiroshima and Nagasaki and of AIDS, a certain social surplus—the reproductively or genetically "impaired" hibakusha, the IV drug user, the person of color, the sex worker, the queer—all those "whose bodies are fetishized as vials of contagion and death," as Linda Singer puts it[49]—is produced in order to maintain liberal humanism's "society," constituted in the genetic, viral, and bacteriological law and order of the clean and proper body, as *the* privileged community of the Same. This social surplus, so-called, is not merely the index of the proliferation of objects before the panoptic Gaze of a magisterial transcendental subjectivity (the social scientist–engineer); much more radically, it is the endless proliferation of difference itself, signifying the radical impossibility of constituting "society" as totality. It is therefore undoubtedly as something other than a humanism that steadfastly refuses to think the apocalyptic ground of its destitution that Ōta Yōko invokes a being-in-common constituted in the entropic indifference of pure difference when she writes, "The somber reminder that we have a common fate absolutely forbids us to indulge in either nihilism or easy evasion" (271). For essential reasons, of course, it would be impossible to say what this something-other-than-a-humanism might be (which would be to ascribe to such a being-in-common a ground). It can become neither the mere outside of humanism, the transcendent beyond of humanism, nor the simply marginal. In *City of Corpses*, it is the figure of she who transgresses boundaries—the figure of the refugee, the gypsy, the nomad—that is the index of the sociality of a being-in-common perversely grounded in destitution.

Immediately after the bombing, the narrator records that "with neither land nor houses of their own, a bunch of nomads had found a bit of land on the edge of a river and were living a rootless existence, one day at a time. That is what the mass of people I saw on the riverbed looked like" (218). The existential destitution of the nomads, that nomadism which is their destitution, becomes an ontological promiscuity, as it were: their existentiality is the indiscriminate punctuality of the whatever, whenever, wherever. Furthermore, their nonplace is that of the outlaw. Looking for food in the countryside, the narrator and her mother and sister "had only two alternatives: beg and whine like gypsies, who cried outside people's houses even when they had in their pockets the money to pay the staggering prices of the black market, or become thieves" (241). Or, again: "We who have come from the outside are all gypsies; we have money but no food" (272). The hibakusha—refugee, nomad, gypsy—thus occupies no place, but is, in her "being," the very movement of transgression itself, the impossibility of being situated within the borders of any ie, domus, habitus, or Heimat, whether construed as village, nation, or what is called the human community. The Jew, the gypsy, the queer: this is what humanism is afraid of—

what humanism *must* be afraid of—in order to constitute itself. For
here is the impossibility of the domesticity of any domus. It is in
the pure relationality of homelessness (figured in *City of Corpses* as
money unattached to any commodity-object), in its essential transgression of constitutive boundaries (such as "life" and "death"), in
the nomadism of the relation of nonrelation, in destitution, that
such a being-in-common must be thought. Chapters 5 and 7 of the
present investigation pursues the question in texts by David Wojnarowicz and Sue Golding. Such a sociality, I am trying to suggest,
must be sought precisely in the passage of the phenomenological
through and as its own impossibility, in its aporiae, which are apocalyptic.

The Itinerary of Withdrawal

City of Corpses also describes the itinerary of an attempted retreat to the plenitude and sufficiency of the community of the domus, a retreat that nevertheless finds a specific impossibility installed
in the innermost recesses of the domesticity of the quotidian. There
are at least five intersecting and strictly coterminous trajectories
here. First, there is a geographical itinerary, a series of secessions
from the center, from the metropolis or even the megalopolis.
Which is, second, at the same time a retreat to the essential domesticity of the rhythmicity of daily life, as in Takenishi. Which, third,
is thereby and as such an archaeology in search of the *archē* of the
cultural as such, ultimately an attempt to repeat the inaugural institution of culture. Fourth, and concomitantly, there is an archaeological interrogation of the historical Imaginary, wherein a suffi-
ciently historicized past is that in relation to which henceforth no
relation of continuity is thinkable; to think any such continuity will
occlude the apocalyptic event of historicity as such. Fifth, and finally, these are at the same time a radical thought of "Japan" as the
impossibility of the accomplishment of community in the communion of an essential inarticulable communication. The possibility
for community will henceforth be disabled by the disclosure, in the

lapsus or syncope of the event, of destitution as the apocalyptic ground of the historico-social.

Now certainly all of this might be thought to be the expression of a certain nostalgia, the nostalgia of homo re-domesticus, one who seeks in historicization the domestication of historicity and sociality. But that evaluation would in the present instance be to ignore the *writing* of *City of Corpses*. Before we come to this question, however, it is necessary to retrace the itineraries I have just sketched.

First, let us consider the geographical itinerary. A narrative trajectory could be reconstituted here, consisting of a series of secessions from the metropolitan and megalopolitan center. In the first instance from Tokyo, the site of career, of change, of exteriority, of contingency—and above all of the firebombings of the spring of 1945—to the interiority of the maternal home in Hiroshima. A retreat to the maternal in at least two senses: insofar as the maternal home in Hiroshima is not the ancestral, paternal estate in the village, and insofar as it is inhabited solely by women—the narrator, her sister and the latter's child, and their mother—it is difficult not to read this as a retreat to maternity or the maternal *as such*. Hiroshima before 6 August 1945 is recollected after the bombing as possessed of a certain self-sufficient plenitude and separation from more extensive social and political entities, "a cheerful city with a good climate, rich in material goods and a good place to live," possessed of its own dialect and with a distinct personality, "in some respects cheerful, but . . . irresponsible and unsociable" (178). This recollection is in part an ethnography, therefore, an anthropological recollection of an irretrievably lost tribe. The young women, many of whom will shortly be charred "beyond recognition," are light tan, tans significantly attributed to the rivers (179–80). The rivers, recollected in a certain lyricism, are possessed of "a serene and unchanging beauty," particularly in winter. All of this is interrupted, of course, one August morning—no need to ask which—when the rivers and riverbeds become the site of the most unspeakable suffering, and of the impossibility of the thought of the domus. The city is remembered to have given off "a southern warmth, a languid and carefree air, due probably to these rivers and to the fact that the city opened like a fan with its handle to the south" (179). Later, from the perspective of the rural village with its avarice, Hiroshima will be recalled fondly, in spite of everything: "One would not have thought that the riverbed and the cemetery and the streets reeking of rotting human flesh were fit for human habitation; but in the country there even came moments when, on looking back, I thought how pure and clean life in those places had been" (243). Hiroshima, then, is recollected as a refuge from destitution, even from the absolute destitution that Hiroshima had itself become. It is in this refuge that, for a time, the narrator lives a comfortable middle-class life, protected, perhaps by a certain forgetting, from the ravages of the war.

On 6 August 1945, all of this, whatever once it was, becomes nothing but recollection. The domesticity of the comfortable house in Hakushima is destroyed, a destruction from which the narrator and her family seek refuge in the riverbed, and thence make their tortuous way to the countryside: "I have come [to the country] driven out of the burnt-out wasteland of a metropolis totally destroyed, a metropolis no longer deserving of the name; I am so utterly weak and wretched that I have lost all touch with that dream that was once so dear to my heart" (154).

The village to which they retreat (and from which mother and sister will attempt a further retreat) is almost completely isolated from the rest of the world, without electricity, newspapers, food deliveries, to such an extent that they hear nothing of what is going on in nearby Hiroshima in mid-September (263–65). The almost autarkic self-sufficiency of the classical domus, in the sufficient plenitude of its patriarchal economy, the organization of a labor, the work of culture, is one in which, as Lyotard says, "The common work is the domus itself, in other words the community. It is the work of a repeated domestication":[50]

> We sank helplessly into feelings we could not express. In the past, our family's ancient house code had stipulated that we take care of the villagers. This assistance involved special bonds, virtually lifelong, second in importance only to the bonds among blood relations. It

included tutoring the young women at the main house, making chests of drawers and crested *kimonos* for people when they got married, listening to the problems of the young men, getting together to celebrate the joys of marriage or to bemoan divorces, organizing celebrations when children were born. But now, having not visited them for many years, we showed up, beggars, reduced to poverty and accursed. We did not beg in so many words, but without their help we would have starved; so it amounted to the same thing. (241–42)

The terms structuring the domus have been reversed; those who had managed a certain domestic economy as the work of culture and community, return, in the wake of the insistence of the existential, as outsiders, gypsies, thieves, the surplus of the production of the domus and community. Those who had stood as guarantors of the domestic, social, and ultimately political orders (and indeed of order altogether), in the first instance through the management of the techniques of daily life, return from the absolute and unremitting destitution and disorder, the essential anarchy of the historico-social, in search of the archē of relationality, to find that they themselves have become the mortal threat, as pure surplus of the nomadic corpse, to that economy, that domus, to order altogether. "We [had] lost the entire property to extravagant living in Father's generation." The Father, absent throughout, no longer figures as he who supports the economy, but as he who, through a certain excessiveness, destroys: the Law is no longer "of the Father," another revelation of the anarchic ground of the Symbolic order. Thus, "The family graveyard was the only thing in the village still belonging to us" (213; see also 261). Thus, we have a certain geographical itinerary: from Tokyo to Hiroshima to the village to the family graveyard. Mother and sister, herself a mother, unable to bear the prospect of mere tenancy—which would in any case be merely a hiatus in their essentially nomadic existence—retreat yet further in an attempt to reinvent the domestic culture of the domus; the narrator remains in the destabilized domus of the village in order to write. And it is her writing that accomplishes the destabilization of the consolations of domesticity altogether.

Second, there is a retreat to the very domesticity of daily life.

"Daily life," according to an entire discourse, which we might thereby designate "ethnographic," is constituted, instituted, inscribed as the nomological (presumptively ontological) regularity of a technical, instrumental relation, expressed in tools and artifacts, in the instrumentality of what is called the body, and in the instrumentality of what is called language, to the things of the world. This "ethnography," in both its formal and informal articulations, frequently takes this relation to be constitutive of the subject/object relation in its particularities, even as it is constituted *by* the subject/object relation. Daily life is thereby constituted for this "ethnography" in the rhythmicity or repetition (custom) of that subject/object instrumental relation (in a nonerotic relation, therefore). The subjectivity of an "I" is either expressed in or emerges from (but in either case is inextricably bound up with) the ways in which (or techniques by means of which) the "I" grasps the things of the world (including the "body" and "language"). This relation may be thought, for example, as use-value, as Brauch, as technological dominance, or as the opposition of culture to nature. But in any case it is thought as the ground of the cultural as such, and therefore of subjectivity as such. This relation has been thought, furthermore, as the ground of the economic as such (the *oikonomia*), of the human, and of differences (race, ethnicity, gender, class, and sexuality, for example) that are thereby thought as cultural differences, and as cultural subjectivities. But in each instance the question of subjectivity is thought in terms of a subject/object relation, and in terms of its nomological, presumptively ontological, regularity—in its continuity and stability—in its forgetting of the absolute destitution of a radical historicity. What, then, of an apocalyptic, which is—precisely—possessed of no quotidian? There is no daily life in hell, or in the hell that was Hiroshima. *City of Corpses* records an irremediable breach in the domestic economy of the domus and of cultural community, revealing the absolute contingency of this instrumental relation; it thereby demands a rethinking of that relation.

In the flash of the explosion, and in the fires of its immediate aftermath, virtually all of the things or objects of the world in relation to which a relation to the world is sustained, the relation that constitutes the material support of subjectivity, are either destroyed outright, so deformed as to be, precisely, useless, or survive bereft of the systematic relations that made them useful or "meaningful" in the first place: they become empty signifiers, signifying only their own nonrelation to any signified—corpses of a psychotic material culture (183). Thus it is only the narrator's mother, she who expresses and safeguards the very domesticity of the domus, who "would keep going back into the house in search of things" (186). The narrator, as we have seen, records her own indifference to the essential indifference of this psychosis of material quotidian culture.

Those who could still move at all made their way before the spreading fires to the riverbeds, a gathering of living corpses in utter physical abjection:

> The stream of people fleeing became constant and unending. The desirable places—for example, the shady spots where one could escape the sun—were soon gone. . . .
> Here and there on the hot sand people were sitting, standing around, or stretched out as if dead. Those with burns vomited continuously, and the sound was nerve-wracking. . . . With people arriving all the while, the human mass on the riverbed grew still larger.
> Quickly locating small places of their own, they settled in.
> No matter what the situation, it seems, people are always impatient to find a place to call their own. Even out-of-doors, people clearly prefer not to be jumbled together but to have exclusive possession of a specific piece of ground. (188–89)

For women on the riverbed, there is an extraordinary relation to what might almost be called the carnivalesque. Throughout their lives, their subjectivities have been defined by service to the domus (constituting thereby its domesticity) in the rhythmic regularity of the economy of labor, in an instrumental relation to the things of the world. But:

> Around us that morning we heard typical morning chitchat. "Well, well. A welcome morning! Nothing to do. I'm forty-one years old, and this is the first time I've had a morning with so little to do!"

There came the sound of light female laughter. "That's how it is when you have a house to run. First thing in the morning to last thing at night—so busy all day you go dizzy. Get up; while it's still dark out, clean the whole house, living room to toilet. Do the cooking. The washing. Mind the children, too. Meanwhile—can't tell when—the delivery man knocks; you run to answer. Get back again; boil and roast—if you've got something to cook, fine. Complain that you haven't this, haven't that; but even while complaining, make do somehow; boil and fry something. But take this morning now. Not a thing to do!" (200)

Surely what is at stake here are the regulative norms of the quotidian, of the economy of daily life that sustains the community of the domus; but what are thereby *also* at stake are the very subjectivities of the women. No housekeeping during the apocalypse. What we witness in the apocalyptic destitution of the riverbed is a desperate attempt, not only to provide what count as "the necessities" of life, but (and this is not merely an implication or effect, but what is happening *in* and *as* the desperation of the struggle) to reconstitute, through a certain "deformed" instrumentality, culture and the community itself: the work of the domus is the domus itself; the "community" cannot be *désoeuvrée*, for madness is the absence of work. What the reconstitution of the quotidian would accomplish, therefore, would be the occlusion of madness, of the anarchic, destitute, apocalyptic ground of the historico-social.

It is all this—the impossible reconstitution of the domus and of subjectivity—that is at stake when it is a matter of eating. Although in Tokyo "the talk of food stopped when the bombing became fierce," because "[l]ife itself is more important than the mundane matter of wanting to eat" (242), what is at stake in the riverbed is not in the first or last instance merely a matter of a certain physiology: it never is. So it is in the (im)possibility of reconstituting the domus and subjectivity through a restored domesticity of the quotidian that resides the source of whatever satisfaction might be gotten from food on the riverbed (194; 221–23).

So it is in an entirely *other* relation that the narrator would think a sociality, a being-in-common grounded in the entropic indifferent pure difference of destitution, *other* than the relation of sameness that constituted the community of the domus:

> That experience of living for three days on the riverbed among all those corpses, horrible as it was, left me as a human being with a profound and unique lesson I shall never forget. Lives hinged on whether one had evacuated to a safe place before August 6. One speaks of the simple life, but I have a sense that now I have grasped its true form. Before, try as I might, I hadn't been able to. . . . My life up until then I had thought of as simple, but I realize I had been wrong. I had had too many possessions; I had been controlled by them; and my very spirit had coarsened. (270)

Here, then, is the thought, however inchoate (and however inchoate it must necessarily be, and however much it may depend on the vocabulary of humanism), that the historico-social, that culture, that what constitutes daily life, and that we designate by the term "daily life," that community, must be thought from an entirely *other* relation than the subject/object relation (or, rather, must always also be thought as the surplus or excess of the subject/object relation), from the thought of a technique that might be other than technology, from the thought of a "culture" that would be a separation, certainly, but an originary separation, a separation that would not be a separation-*from* ("nature"): which would be to think culture as historicity.

Third, there is in *City of Corpses* an itinerary that becomes an archaeology of the material culture of daily life:

> I walked along the rubble-strewn street, still warm, to the spot in front of our house. When I saw Mother, my tears stopped of their own accord. The house had burned so completely one could not imagine that a house had ever stood there. Two stone gateposts remained, protruding from the ground like cemetery headstones; where the bath had been, only the metal tub remained, scorched a rust color and looking unreal. In addition, the frame of the sewing machine that had been on the second floor, the shears that had been at the bottom of the parcel to go to the country, and two or three pieces of pottery were half-buried in the burned ground, reduced to ash though still holding their shape. Mother and I exchanged a silent glance.

Then Mother said, "What do you suppose happened to all the glass? There aren't even any broken bits!"

Indeed, the glass was gone without a trace. Perhaps, melted down like jelly, it had flowed away? As for the pots and kettles, some-one might have stolen them in the last three days, so people said; but I thought they too might have melted down and flowed away. We also saw ashes in the shape of the wicker trunk, ashes in the shape of the camera bag, and so on.

At the air raid shelter in the cemetery, the four or five thick quilts Mother had thrown into the entrance as she left were gone; only a mound of ashes was left. Some time ago we had placed a sturdy box filled with foodstuffs in the front half of the shelter; that large box had acted as a wall, and the things beyond it had not burned.

What had not burned? The portable charcoal stove and the pots and kettles and a scant three trunks of clothing. When I saw the things that hadn't burned, I felt as I would feel on seeing, safe and sound, people I thought had died: how wonderful to clasp their hands in mine! The pots and kettles and trunks seemed to be calling out to us; it irritated me that they didn't come walking out toward us now of their own accord. (219–20)

We are presented here with a specifically *archaeological* scene of the re-mains of a material quotidian culture, the ruin of the domus. There is nothing here that would differentiate between the most ancient foun-dations uncovered in a formal dig and the detritus of the day before yesterday; there is no distinction here between a virtually immemor-ial distant past and the present. This archaeology, therefore, does not attempt to reconstitute a continuity in the name of the origin of cul-ture such as would, in the regularity and rhythmicity of quotidian custom, establish a continuity as the repetition of an inaugural found-ing moment. Rather, it renders the present of the domus—its use values, its conjunction of use and need, its sufficiency and plenitude, its culture and subjectivity—an irrecoverable prehistory, the traces (ashes, cinders) of an untranscendable difference. We are presented with the utter strangeness and distance of what is most near, the ab-solute inaccessibility of what is at hand. As if one were suddenly to find oneself the only native speaker of a long extinct language, or to find one's "own" body to be that of the embalmed Osiris.

What is at stake here is not the work of mourning (or that work of mourning which would be culture, which makes sense of the past), for although the work of mourning ostensibly insists upon a recognition of the pastness of the past, it does so in establishing a continuity with the past, in a working through, a presentification of the past that becomes thereby a past that, in Dennis Schmidt's lapidary phrase, "had no other future than us."[51] Rather, in this archaeology, the past becomes an absence with which the present essentially cannot communicate. This archaeology therefore bespeaks a radical historicity. Here it is the very familiarity of everyday life that becomes itself the untranscendable alterity of an irrecoverable past; no longer can the artifacts—*hibachi*, pots and kettles, trunks of clothes—call the narrator to subjectivity in the interpellation she imagines: "it irritated me that they didn't come walking toward us of their own accord." These artifacts become those museum pieces simply labeled "stone implement" or "clay pot," forever bereft of any relation to the *Erlebnis* of their usage; they become the traces of irretrievably lost quotidian practices, practices that would constitute the cultural domus as such. This archaeology in search of the archē of the culture of the domus finds merely the traces of destitution, leaving one bereft of any technē that would enable a being-in-the-world. "Culture" thereby becomes not merely separation (from "nature," for example), but designates the fact of an originary separation "before" any imagined unity, the fact of separation "itself," a nonidentity that is the ground of identity. Archaeology here is the impossibility of the achievement of any historicization, and of any identification in the historical Imaginary (as Bildung, for example). This archaeology reveals at least an isomorphic relation between historicization and domestication, and this precisely in revealing the impossibility of domesticating or historicizing historicity. The historical Imaginary becomes something quite other than the site of a specular identification; it becomes the impossibility of such an identification. Here, "historicity" indicates the essential absence of specularity. In the time of AIDS, we are all of us vampires: the insistence of the existential has seen to that. (Of course, this impossibility of specular identification must always figure as the *surplus* of specularity, identification, historicization.)

The Historical Itinerary

The historical Imaginary that is invoked in, and that is the support of, the large majority of appeals to "historical consciousness," "history itself," or simply History, is, we know very well, the site of an identification that is *presumptively* a *specular* identification. In the mirror of history, we are told, we find our ownmost proper identity. This identification is not necessarily with the heroic figure, or with a group or subgroup, or even in the disavowal of such an identification. Often enough, it is an identification with the quotidian banality of a technique, or technical/technological practice, of a relation to the things of the world; an identification with an instrumental relation (to the body, to language, to things, to the practices of their deployment in negotiations with what we call the world), which instrumental relation is constitutive of the community (i.e., the economy) of the domus. This is particularly obvious in the instance of national histories (or histories of any community, whatever their other differences), but no less so in the instances of cultural, social, economic, and intellectual historiographies. The identification is not necessarily in the first instance with the identity of the actor(s), nor even with what is done, but with the technique by which some practice is enacted. This identification is frequently presented, under the rubrics of "human nature" or "our common humanity," or of the commonality of any community, as a simple, straightforward specularity. Such a historiography says "thou art that," but only because "that" has always already been "thou."

Such were the deployments of historiography, albeit at a very crude, propagandistic level, by the government in wartime Japan (as with any number of other patriotisms, of course): "In society at large people were still preaching the patriotic zeal of Kusunoki Masashige. The ancient etiquette of the battlefield called for individual combat between mounted knights, each of whom announced his name and fought gloriously" (210). A historical Imaginary as old, but no older, than the *Heike monogatari* itself. Here the ideological interpellation of the Imaginary subject is quite explicit: in identifying with Kusunoki Masashige (or "samurai of old"), you will come to the same subjectivity on the battlefield as they; it is in fact an identify that has, as a good Japanese, always been yours; your identity is accomplished in your death. At any literal level, this is a crude ploy indeed, but in its *logic*, as we saw in reading Nishida, persuasive and effective. Encoded as fate, destiny, tragedy, a certain comportment (which is to say, a certain instrumental relation, a certain technique) is the guarantor of a belonging to the culture, the *gathering*, which is the community of the domus. But, the narrator notes, "It makes no sense to think of waging modern war for ten or even fifteen years, [with] etiquette [which is to say, a technique] as proper as with the samurai of old [and that made a samurai in fact a samurai], in leisurely fashion" (165). There is an awareness here of the radical impossibility of any specular identification in the historical Imaginary; by virtue of the insistence of the existential (a technological "modern warfare" that achieves its apotheosis in the apocalypse of Hiroshima and Nagasaki), by virtue of the nondiscrimination, the indifference of pure difference, the infinite punctuality of the event, it becomes impossible to think the ideological continuity between that particular historical Imaginary and the present situation (it becomes impossible to identify, that is to say).

Moreover, and far more radically, it becomes henceforth impossible to think the historical Imaginary to be the site of any possible identification (even as inverse disavowal). The historical Imaginary is no longer the site at which the similitude of the community of the domus is accomplished, but rather the site of its impossibility. After 8:15:17 A.M. on 6 August 1945, the past has passed—something we have still to learn. Thus, the historical Imaginary is henceforth the site of a certain impossibility; the image of the past will no longer figure in every historiography, formal or informal, as the security of the domus to which one might return, even in rueful nostalgia. Rather, it will serve as the image of the archaeological revelation of the essentially imaginary nature of the plenitude and sufficiency of the domus (and the past as domus), a revelation of the historicity or destitution of what is. Henceforth, the image of the past will be one of the impossibility of domestication. Thus, when the narrator recalls the Hiroshima of "before" (and, as in the case of

AIDS diagnoses, it will never any longer be necessary to wonder "before what?")—the Hiroshima that was once the domus of the Asano, whose castle town it was; the domus that lived in the shadow of neighboring Chōshū (178)—when she mourns the great white castle of the Asano, which "looked as if it had collapsed and shattered without offering much resistance," she recognizes that "[e]ven supposing a new city were to be built on this land, there would be no rebuilding the castle" (226).

"Hiroshima was a flat city with no hills. Thanks to its white castle, Hiroshima became three-dimensional and preserved the flavor of the past. Hiroshima, too, had its history, and it saddened me to march forward over the corpse of the past" (226). This is a nostalgia, certainly, for the image of an obliterated possibility for domestic community, but also, and *thereby*, a nostalgia for the domus of history, for history-as-domus. "History" becomes the Doppelgänger of every invocation of history, forevermore the index of the apocalypse that the historical Imaginary occludes.

The Geopolitical Itinerary

The figure of "Japan" is undoubtedly inscribed in numerous, overdetermined, ambiguous, and even contradictory ways in *City of Corpses*. Of these, two are especially pertinent to the present investigation. First, "Japan" figures as a cultural and economic domus; second, "Japan," which both is and is not the "Japan" of a domestic culture, also figures as a geopolitical entity.

The ideological construction of "Japan" as a domestic culture of the domus is by now well known; this construction is certainly not limited to "Japan," nor did it end in the postwar period. Indeed, it persists both in the popular culture as *Nihonjinron* as well as in formal academic discourse. In the forms of state propaganda in the 1930's and 1940's, it frequently quite specifically relied upon a conception of the ie (or domus) construed as what social science would call an extended family, in which the figure of the emperor was quite specifically *maternal*. But it must be understood that these relatively crude, albeit effective, formulations emerged from, even as they trivialized, a much more profound cultural criticism, in which the term "culture" marked the site of a disturbing questioning. One thinks of those for whom the thematics of the present essay would have been not at all alien—Nishida Kitarō, Miki Kiyoshi, Watsuji Tetsurō, Tanabe Hajime, Tanizaki Jun'ichirō, Kobayashi Hideo, Tosaka Jun—for example. In the postwar period, what had been a questioning in the first half of the century has become a series of unthought commonplaces, in Japan as elsewhere. Nowhere is this more readily apparent than in the collusion of a cultural essentialism with a liberal internationalist humanism. One only has to think of the purposes to which the annual memorial services at Hiroshima and Nagasaki have been put, or of government policy regarding AIDS in the early years of the pandemic, when national boundaries were thought to provide some measure of what Asada Akira has called "cultural inoculation."[52] What all this amounts to is the occlusion of the apocalyptic.

When *City of Corpses* reflects upon and offers a characterology of the Japanese, it is, whether intentionally or not, an intervention in the ideological construction of the cultural, economic, domestic *ethnos*. When, for example, the narrator says that, "even before the atomic bombs, Japan itself had already fallen to the mental state epitomized by expressionless faces" (169), when she writes that throughout the war it had been impossible to be true to oneself, and that the Japanese "had lost complete the ability to hear, to see, to speak," and that therefore questions of any justification of the war were at best irrelevant (210–11), when she denounces the callous treatment of the hibakusha (235), when she says that the Japanese are essentially shallow, with no depth such as would make them "democratic" (270–71), and thus calls for a radical revolution in thinking, "Japan" has become the very sign of the impossibility of that suturing of the social that is the cultural domus. Here, the alternative would most vociferously *not* be the liberal adjudication of conflicting interests in the public sphere, but a "rethinking" of the very ground of sociality in destitution.

Here there is a recognition that, however "local" or containable the event of Hiroshima, or indeed, "modern warfare," may appear to be, it cannot in fact be encoded as a tragedy, fate, or destiny that befalls the domestic economy of an ethnos; rather, what is at stake is the status of the domus as such, of domesticity and its cultural economy; here there is the acknowledgment of the global or the ecological as the principle of noncontainment (rather than as the concept of totality). In other words, this principle of noncontainment is the guarantee of the infinite proliferation of difference, a principle of surplus or excess; it is the noncontainment indicated in Ōta's invocation of the "common fate" that precludes both "nihilism" and "easy evasion" (271). This noncontainment, this impossibility of suturing the social, as the global or the ecological, means that when the question of "responsibility" is invoked with regard to the war or the bombings of Hiroshima and Nagasaki, the presuppositions of a normative geopolitical historiography are quite simply irrelevant, and in their irrelevance obscure the globality or ecology of the apocalyptic event. Who, indeed, would be responsible for the end of the world? The continual, and continually frustrated, attempts in *City of Corpses* to understand and master the event of 6 August 1945 according to the epistemological protocols—the *categories* in the strong sense of the term—of a normative historiography, in fact witness to the essential incapacity of such a historiography (most particularly when it calls itself "world history") to think the essential noncontainment of the apocalyptic, to think the transgression of limits, to think the impossibilities of thought.

To think, for example, the state-form as such is necessarily—in the aftermath of "Hiroshima"—to think the end, the bankruptcy, of modern political thought. For what is at stake is a power, a technological capacity, which is in principle and in effect *illimitable*. The narrator of *City of Corpses*, perhaps more than Ōta Yōko knew, approached the thought of the unthinkability of the illimitable in her "childish" meditations on the nonrelation of the event to the war, and on the "cosmic," eschatological dimensions of the war (185, 192, 211), as well as in the frustration of her attempt to speculate the elements (249), and in her observation that "[a]ll these effects arose from the fact that such an event had never happened before. A special quality of the damage the atomic bomb inflicts lies in the extreme unease it generates, unease because the truth is not likely to be known for many years" (177). (And although, of course, we know more, or at least think we do, about the bomb fifty years on, we should not thereby assume that our itinerary has brought us to the truth.)

It is this illimitability, noncontainability, globality, or ecology that "modern political thought" has, by and large and for essential reasons, not thought. Antonio Negri is perhaps one of the very few political theorists who has, however briefly, indicated the dimensions of a consequent thinking of contemporary political forms (principally the state) in the wake of Hiroshima and Nagasaki. Negri has argued that there is an essential discontinuity between the classical modern state-form, however Hobbesian it may have been, and the "nuclear state." Here it is a question, of course, not so much of *which* state possesses a nuclear capability, but that the state-form *as such* is possessed of the resources for nuclear annihilation, an apocalyptic capability. The classical modern state-form exercised sovereignty with respect to the political will of the governed (however brutal, aberrant, or unresponsive that sovereignty may have been to the political will), it had to legitimate its power *in* the relation to the political will of the governed and could always be opposed in a material revolutionary insurgency. The "nuclear state" is, however, the state-form as that which can exercise illimitable power, and is thereby in principle unopposable. There had always been some material limit to the classical modern state; for the nuclear state, there are no limits. Thus the sovereignty of the nuclear state does not resides in legitimation, which might always be withdrawn. The nuclear state *as such* seeks no legitimation from the political will. The sovereignty of the nuclear state resides in the "pure image of power," in the ability to project (and realize) a Doomsday Imaginary. The power, authority, and sovereignty of the nuclear state reside in its ability to engineer the apocalypse. This transition from the classical modern state to the nuclear state is enabled by the secrecy of its operations—the impossibility of witnessing or testifying to them—for reasons of what is, cynically enough, called "national security." Thus, the nuclear state is in essence and in effect, terrorist; fear and terror have become the "basic form of human association." This constitutes what Negri calls the "social capital" of the nuclear state. Now the problem is, as Negri emphasizes, that this "pure image of power," or Doomsday Imaginary, is the self-representation of a state-form against which any resistance is at best futile (the problem, indeed, of any thought of apocalypse).[53]

But the fact that the Doomsday Imaginary serves the interests of the nuclear state should not obscure from view the fact that an apocalyptic Armageddon is technologically feasible, nor that the nuclear state has quite successfully projected an image of itself as the sole possible defense against the terror that it in fact *is*. The conjunction of a technological capability with the projection of an apocalyptic Armageddon (against which the nuclear state projects itself as the sole defense) has a number of effects.

The nuclear state, in essence and in effect terrorist, enforces a recognition of terror as the "ontological" condition. It is essential to the terror of every terrorism that it is radically contingent, that it is "promiscuous," that its time be that of an infinite punctuality and that it escapes any essential determinative causality—it is possible but not predictable at any place and any time, and that its effects are *incalculable* (as in the symptomology of radiation sickness or AIDS). In this sense, terror is the *limit* of every regularity, of every regulative norm, of every possible *nomos*, of the Law, indeed the lo-gos, *as such*. The terror in the hands of the nuclear state renders impossible any *justification* of the ethico-political. Because this terror is absolute or illimitable, it usurps the place so long reserved for God, that other terrorist. In the time of the nuclear state, power *is* this radical unjustifiability of the exercise of power: there can be no rationality that authorizes or warrants the use or deployment of a nuclear capability. Contradictorily, the institutionalized terrorism that is the nuclear state is, in this sense, anarchic. And this anarchy is what must henceforth count as the ground of historico-social being. Thus, there can be no teratology or phenomenology (or indeed, onto-theology) adequate to the thought of this terror. And political thought has yet to think this insufficiency as its ground.

Furthermore, nuclear terror is global or ecological, not merely because of the devastation it brings to what is called the environment, but because it is in principle illimitable, saturating what is, without limit, without boundaries, and *therefore* without any possible prophylaxis. (Nuclear-free zones are, as we know, a pleasant but vacuous and dangerous fantasy.) This thought of the global or the ecological is the thought of the first (and last) actualization, in its annihilation, of totality. Every place becomes the site of destitution: the terrorism of the nuclear state resides in the fact that it is possessed of no outside.

Which means, taken together, that what the nuclear state, in its projection of apocalypse and as institutionalized terrorism, *does*, is transform all of us, always already, into "victims," the abject objects of a proleptic work of mourning. Thus we are rendered essentially passive, utterly deprived of any agency, any possibility for consequent action. The ultimate entropy of destitution renders us immobile. But what if to come to this conclusion is too easily to conflate agency with subjectivity? What if the only possibility for consequent intervention resided in the nonpositive affirmation of our destitution? What if that possibility were to reside in the affirmation of the anarchy, the groundlessness, of the historico-social? In "going to ground"? Certainly this would concomitantly require another thought of the relation to "things," to sociality, and to the ethico-political, a thought that could only proceed from the unthinkability of the anarchic ground of an absolute destitution. The subsequent essays of this investigation pursue such possibilities.

But such thinking would also require a reflection on the writing of *City of Corpses*.

The Itinerary of a Writing

The first chapter of *City of Corpses*, "An Autumn So Horrible Even the Stones Cry Out," opens with an evocation of the infinite punctuality, the whenever, the whatever, of the destitution of the apocalyptic. "I have always wanted to spend an autumn in the country," the narrator acknowledges, but driven from the metropolis (first Tokyo, then Hiroshima), she finds that she is "so utterly weak and wretched that I have lost all touch with that dream that was once so dear to my heart" (153–54). There follows a lyrical description of a rural autumn landscape, ostensibly drawn from "memories of childhood": "Even in the midst of Tokyo, where life was often unkind, such memories of the landscape revived me. In Tokyo I often thought: some day I'll go back to that place of my memories and take a long vacation" (154). But:

> Now I have come at last to the countryside of which I was so fond. Afflicted in body and soul by the brutality of war, I have come to lay my body down. I look at the light purple mountains, at the perfectly blue sky; at night I sit looking at the brilliance of the moon or listening to the sound of flowing water. But those sights and sounds no longer hold me spellbound. (154)

What we are apparently witnessing in this and a number of comparable passages is the memory of—and present aspiration to—an overcoming or transcendence of the separation that maintains the difference between the ultimate plenitude of "nature" and the fragmentation, difference, and dispersions of culture, a nostalgia for the integration and indifferent solace of the outside of technique, language, culture, history, and historicity, a nostalgia for an ultimate domesticity. Perhaps, indeed, these passages mark a nostalgia for the imaginary ontological plenitude of an "outside" of historicity. But if so, this nostalgia is first of all a nostalgia, not for "nature" altogether, but for a *landscape*, a landscape that situates she who sees within, but also beyond, a certain perspective as the possessor of the Gaze, thereby positioning she who sees in the place of a transcendental subject, a Gaze that puts things, as historians are wont to say, "in perspective," but a perspective that exists in fact only in its positioning of a meditative subject.[54] What is encoded here as nostalgia for a putatively lost transcendental plenitude or ontological sufficiency is perhaps, more to the point, the memory of a *seduction* by the "sights and sounds" of a specifically *literary* landscape—indeed, the landscape of the literary as such, or of literariness per se. What is no longer desirable or seductive here is that very literariness, a literary landscape that in certain formulations is at least as old as the *Genji monogatari.* Thus, for example, "The voices of insects, too, came to our ears. It was all so very sad" (196). But there are insects other than these literary insects about:

> A full month after August 6, people said, corpses lay wherever you went in the city, skeletons were everywhere, and a nauseating smell blanketed the city. Flies were all over the place, as if someone had scattered red beans; the flies were so dense in the burned streetcars running in some parts of the city that they turned the passengers' skin pitch black; big black flies swarmed hideously, particularly on the faces of babies. Flies even got inside those aluminum lunch boxes with the tight lids and expired atop the rice. (265; see also 206)

Certainly the memory of the seduction that is literariness—or "art"—haunts the text of *City of Corpses* throughout; but whatever might once have been the case, that seduction has lost all its attractions, however fatal; its "sights and sounds no longer hold me spellbound," the literary object can no longer hold the fascinated Gaze of the subject in the luminosity of its transcendence. As an effect of the insistence of the existential—a zero-degree *aisthēsis*—the aesthetic, be it of the sublime *or* of the beautiful—fails, and fails *radically.* (Here it must be emphasized that it is also a failure of any aesthetic of the sublime; the apocalypse is not a Götterdämmerung.) The literary fails in the absolute nontranscendence, the utter destitution, of what is; there can be no aesthetics of meaning here. Lost is the hope that out of great suffering might come an art that would be the transcendence of that suffering, and that would do so in making that suffering in some sense meaningful; such a transcendence could only consist of a donation of meaning.

Thus, in the preface to the second edition (1950), the first uncensored edition, Ōta Yōko records the impossibility of an adequate and sufficient literary treatment of what happened at Hiroshima, the failure of the seduction of the literary as such. Our question is, What is at stake when it is the seduction of the literary that is at stake?

In the first instance, Ōta claims that the literary insufficiency of *City of Corpses* is the effect of a certain material and intractable urgency; writing between August and November of 1945, Ōta "was living at the time on a razor's edge between life and death, never knowing from moment to moment when death would drag me over to its side," and therefore, "had no time to organize *City of Corpses* in good literary form. . . . in the format of superior fiction" (147), resulting in "a concrete piece of writing that was something less than literature" (150). Writing from within the chasm that separates (and in separating also brings together and sustains the binary opposition of) life and death, this writing can therefore never be merely a writing *about*, the trace of a subject contemplating an object. And it is for this reason that it is ultimately as impossible to contextualize and historicize *City of Corpses* as much as it is a failure of *City of Corpses* to historicize and contextualize that of which it speaks. The writing of *City of Corpses* is very much what the writing of *City of Corpses* is writing *about*; *about* the very *(im)possibility* of any writing whatsoever; something more than a mere reflexivity or reflection is at stake here. Or rather, *City of Corpses* demonstrates what is at stake when it is reflexivity or self-reflection that is at stake.

But at the same time, Ōta writes about the necessary and radical insufficiency of the literary as such:

> [S]urprisingly enough, the city of death that the dropping of the atomic bomb on Hiroshima created makes very difficult subject matter for literature. The new methods of description and expression necessary to write cannot be found in the repertoire of an established writer. I have not seen hell, nor do I acknowledge the existence of the Buddhist hell. Losing sight of the exaggeration involved, people often spoke of the experience of the atomic bomb as "hell" or "scenes of hell." It would probably have been a simple matter if one were able to express the bitterness of that experience in terms of that ready-made concept "hell," whose existence I did not acknowledge. I was absolutely unable to depict the truth without first creating a new terminology. (148)

Indeed, it is a failure of representation in general: "Try as one might to depict that in writing, it cannot be done" (149).

So here, apparently, *in* and *as* the writing of *City of Corpses*, representation and the literary meet their limit, the limit that is also their innermost possibility, a limit, a possibility (for coherence, experience, understanding, meaning) that resides in the chiasmic syncope *between* life and death, *between* madness and sense, *between* transcendence and destitution. It is first of all a matter of witnessing, of testimony to that for which the vocabulary of horror is utterly and essentially insufficient. Between life and death, there is an irrecusable demand for witness, for testimony:

> On this street there were corpses lying on the right, on the left, and even in the middle of the road. The corpses were all headed in the direction of the hospital, some face up, some face down. Eyes and mouths all swollen shut and limbs, too, as swollen as they could possibly be, they looked like huge ugly rubber balls. Even as I wept, I engraved the appearance of these people on my heart.
> "You're really looking at them—how can you? I can't stand and look at corpses." Sister seemed to be criticizing me. I replied, "I'm looking with two sets of eyes—the eyes of a human being and the eyes of a writer."
> "Can you write—about something like this?"
> "Some day I'll have to. That's the responsibility of a writer who's seen it." (205)

At least two major thematics are opened up, and converge, in this passage, and it is the convergence of the thematics of witnessing, testimony, and the imperative that compels the narrator to witness and testify *with* a thematics of writing, and above all *this* writing *as* limit-experience, that is most problematic for any conception of the possibility for transcendence. In other words, we are confronted with the convergence of an imperative zero-degree historiography *with* the historicity of the possibility for the historiographical *as such*.

From all that has been said in this reading of Takenishi and Ōta, it is clear that any notion of witnessing or testimony along the lines of a naive empiricism or positivism, in which representation is held to be at least ideally adequate to its object as a relation of correspondence, is impossible. Rather, we are dealing with a *radical* empiricism in which the event in its incommensurable singularity is, seriously, unthinkable, unrepresentable, unimaginable, unspeakable, and unbearable. In other words, absent for consciousness and representation. The theme has been explored, after all, by Gilles Deleuze, by Lyotard, and by Felman and Laub at great length. And if we recall that it is after all some notion of witnessing or testimony that is necessarily the zero degree of any historiographical practice, then any notion of historiography that relies upon the immediate legibility and transparence of the event is essentially compromised. It would therefore seem that the event could never be the object of an intuition; an object, an intuition that would authorize or provide an epistemological warrant for a historiographical practice. What, then, would be the status of the intuition of the intuition of *that* aporia? What here would be the status of the insistence of the existential, the force of the Outside? Is this necessarily "merely" (as if there were anything mere about it) an "enabling fiction"? Is the originary ground of historical consciousness and of historiography also its end game?

If witnessing or testimony is conceived solely in terms of representation and the relation to the object of representation, then clearly our questions could only be concerned with epistemological validity, with questions of verification, correspondence, adequation, hermeneutic circles (vicious and otherwise), and so forth. But if it is not merely a question of representation and truth debated among various candidates for a chair in transcendental subjectivity, searching in vain for the ground upon which the *différend* could be adjudicated, then we are confronted with a rather more unsettling and disturbing questioning. For what would be at stake is not really the adequacy of what is said to that of which something is said, but of the very possibility of speaking at all. As both Lyotard and Felman and Laub have seen, the witness who testifies first of all testifies to her witnessing; she first of all witnesses that she is a witness, and testifies, *in* testifying to whatever else she testifies to, *to the fact that she testifies*. What she says, her representations, can of course be challenged, verified, and subjected to all kinds of epistemological protocols, for she may, after all, be mad, or lying. What is indisputable, however, is that she witnesses to her witness, testifies to the fact that she testifies. Now this "speech act" is radically—essentially—indeterminable: for, as Nishida once argued, there can be no logical proof of the existence of the self. In this respect, witnessing and testimony are constituted outside of the epistemological and can never be recuperated for meaning and knowing (which is why this is no simple claim, Cartesian or otherwise, to self-presence). Witnessing and testimony are in this respect essentially and necessarily *unjustifiable*, precisely because the existence of the self, in its incommensurable singularity, is radically unjustifiable. This is to take empiricism to its limit, and its limit is, precisely, the insistence of the existential. Hence, every witnessing must be, in the very *act* of witnessing to whatever it is that is being witnessed to, a witnessing to the impossibility of witnessing; every testimony testifies to the impossibility of testimony. Every witnessing must be, as Laub says, a stammering, a speech that testifies to the impossibility of the speaking that is in fact being spoken. Here, testimony (or the writing of *City of Corpses*) *is* not merely, or even first of all, a representation *of* the limit-experience, but *is* in fact the limit-experience, the experience of the limits of experience, the experience of the limit at which experience and testimony are surpassed, the experience of the experiential aporia, the surplus or beyond of experience.

Thus the question of the imperative that demands this witnessing, the question of whence this exigency comes, is—most seriously—absurd. It can be conceived as an—*the*—ethical responsibility imposed as coming from the Other, or from others, or from God, or from a Third. What matters is that this imperative, this call (which is at the same time a scream of abject terror) is the index of the originary unjustifiability or anarchy of the ethico-political dimension. What matters is that the ethico-political exigency of witnessing and testimony remains a *question*. This stammering (a speech that is the impossibility of speaking, an impossibility of speaking that is *thereby* a speaking, all of which is the writing of *City of Corpses*) is untranscendable; there can be no redemption into meaning, historiography, contextuality, art, or "literature." Any answer to the question of the ground of the ethico-political (i.e., why and whence the exigency of witnessing and testimony?) evacuates the ethico-political of any possibility whatsoever for actualization. Any possibility for the ethico-political depends upon this singular unsurpassable stuttering.[55]

But let us attend a bit more closely to the second thematics of the passage, that of writing as limit-experience, a limit-experience that is at the heart of testimony and hence of the historiographical. Here let me offer a formula, derived from reading Blanchot and Fynsk, in a vocabulary appropriated from Fynsk: Writing, and the writing that is *City of Corpses*, is the nonrelating relation—or the relation of nonrelation—between the image of pure surplus, the corpse, and the sheer improbability of the fact that "there is" language, the fact of the possibility for sense or meaning at all, the fact of the "il y a" or "Es gibt" of language, thought, and history. This relation of nonrelation is the limit-experience of writing.

In the passage quoted above, the narrator's sister ostensibly refuses her fascination with the image of the corpses (although it could of course be argued that that refusal to see the corpses is precisely the index of an intense fascination). The narrator, however, feels obliged (and it is the nature of this obligation that concerns us) to see with two sets of eyes—those of a human being and those of a writer. A "writer," then, is something more perhaps, something less perhaps, but in any case something other than a "human being"—she will see and write from outside the closure of an intersubjective recognition, outside "humanism." It is not merely the "human being" who will witness and testify, but the "writer." And it is *as* a "writer" that she is fascinated by the image of the corpses; perhaps it is her fascination with the image of the corpses that makes of a human being that also-something-other-than-human that is a "writer." In any case, a certain disjunct simultaneity of "seeing" (witnessing) and "writing" (testimony) constitutes her "responsibility," the imperative to "write." And it is not simply a matter of transposing seeing into writing, of translating a certain visibility into a certain comprehensibility. Indeed, it is the very untranslatability of the image into the word, a nonrelation therefore, that is at stake here. The image of the corpses—the image that the corpses *are*—if it is an image *of* anything, is an image of pure surplus, or rather image *as* pure surplus (the nonreferentiality of the singularity of the individual thing in its materiality): the corpse, as Blanchot notes, is not the image of the life that once inhabited it: life sinks into its image. *The image does not communicate with the word*, and the word "corpse" signals this noncommunication. The word "corpse" is in this sense not a reference except to the impossibility of reference, the noncommunication of image and word. Thus the word "corpse" is the corpse of the world "corpse." The word "corpse" is possessed of a corpse-like materiality. (If you write "your own" name often enough, it appears as a pure, nonreferential, image; in other words it becomes a pure image with no reference, no relation, to "you.") In the cases of both the image that the corpse is, and the image of "corpse" (the material figurality of language bereft of significance and meaning), two "cases" of the impossibility of translation or communication, what is signified is not merely an absent presence, or the absence of presence, or the presence of the absence of presence, but the "sheer improbability" (Fynsk) of the "there is" (the "il y a," the "Es gibt") of language—the improbability of the (im)possibility of communication. If language could not retreat from meaning and signification into its mere material figurality, its noncommunication, its entropy and the destitution of the indifference of pure difference, then there would be no possibility of meaning and signification. In this "retreat" into its materiality, language speaks of nothing except the "pure power of signification." This utter nonrelationality of image and word is the "condition of possibility" for all relationality. In other words, this nonrelation *is* the relation; the relation is the relation of nonrelation (for if it were simply nonrelation it would be altogether impossible to speak, to witness or testify to, nonrelation). To speak of the corpse is to speak of the impossibility of speaking of corpses; but it is also to speak of the impossibility of speaking.

But to speak of the impossibility of speaking of corpses is to speak of corpses; to speak of the impossibility of speaking is to speak. It is only possible to speak of corpses if (and only if) one is thereby speaking of the impossibility of speaking of corpses and of the impossibility of speaking; witnessing or testimony is possibly only if *in* witnessing

or testifying one witnesses or testifies to the impossibility of witnessing or testimony. What the narrator of *City of Corpses* calls a
"human being" (her sister, for example, but also that "human being" the narrator *also* is) can neither witness nor testify; "the human" here, then, is constituted in *non*communication, the destitution of the indifference of the pure difference of material singularity. It is the "writer" who "experiences" language as corpse, as the
inhuman, and who experiences writing as death, who can witness
and testify; but she does so only in giving herself to, or in exceeding
herself in, the mute figurality of a language that does not communicate, in the mute figurality of language as nontranscendence.

In this sense, whatever sense or transcendence the literary or
the historiographical may offer is rooted in the senseless nontranscendence of the insistence of the existential, the force of the Outside. Witnessing or testimony—writing—becomes not a record or
representation *of* the insistence of the existential—a *response*—but a
technique: an erotics—of an engagement with the insistence of the
existential without result, which is radically désoeuvrée, which is
in fact an *unworking*, a refusal of the domestic consolations of culture
and knowing, of laying bare its absence-of-ground, of an engagement with the historicity that is its impossible ground. Such is the
sole possibility for historical writing after 6 August 1945. This is the
writing of *City of Corpses*.

Without Justification

A number of figures haunt *City of Corpses*, one of whom is
Gin-chan, who figures in one of the tableaux of the first chapter
and returns, a true revenant, on the last pages. A distant relative of
the narrator's, Gin-chan was a twenty-three-year-old "young
tough," who caused his parents grief and would have been "better
off dead." He led a "bold life," traveling during the war and living in
an illicit relationship with a woman from Kagoshima, with whom
he was in bed when the bomb fell. Having "gone bad at an early
age," he counts for the family as "a juvenile delinquent impossible to

control." A nomad, irresponsible, unaccountably outlaw, within the domestic economy of the ie Gin-chan figures as pure social surplus, given over to nonproductive pleasures, living an unjustified existence.

He first appears slumped in physical abjection on the floor of the house whither the narrator had first retreated after the bombing. Physically, he is beset by radiation sickness, his symptoms already closely resembling those of full-blown AIDS:

> [H]is hair was falling out, and his teeth were loose in his gums as if he had pyorrhea; what is more, he had lost so much weight he was a living skeleton. What stunned me so was the indescribably eerie color of his skin. The skin all over his body was like that of someone in the last stages of tuberculosis, and that color had been painted over with a more hopeless color, opaque like that of roasted eggplant.
>
> The skin around his eyes was tinted lightly, as if tattooed blue; his lips were ashen and dry. His hair was as thin as that of an eighty-year-old and had turned the color of ash. His body was encrusted all over with spots—pale blue, purple, dark blue—the size of beans. (158)

Gin-chan releases himself (which is perhaps something other than resignation) to his destitution and abjection: "It's all over with me. I might as well die. Three doctors all told me so." To which the narrator responds, "Tell yourself you are going to live no matter what. Be tough" (159). In short, his case is hopeless; but on the last pages of *City of Corpses*, Gin-chan's "face is still as ghastly as if he were on his deathbed, but he leads a bold life" (273). He is one of those "living corpses" (and thus, literally haunts the writing of *City of Corpses*) who live "by sheer force of will" (273), whose existence itself is without justification, without ground, without meaning or sense. Gin-chan figures, then, as the useless existence of the destitute, outside the Law (the Law of a medical science that decrees death). And he refuses a proleptic work of mourning in his "bold life." But perhaps it is this very embrace of historicity and of a lawless sociality, of the unjustifiability of the *ipse* in its singularity—that "sheer force of will" that makes it possible for Gin-chan to lead "a bold life" in spite of everything.

In Gin-chan, then, is a figure for Chapters 5 and 7, where in readings of David Wojnarowicz and Sue Golding, I take up the thought of the historico-social, and thereby a politics of inconsolable perversity, from the anarchic ground of apocalyptic destitution. It is a matter, *the* matter in the first instance, of the surplus of a certain technique, a surplus that might be the erotic, a technique that produces no work.

CHAPTER 5

Y Su Sangre Ya Viene Cantando

The somber reminder that we have a common fate absolutely
forbids us to indulge in either nihilism or easy evasion.

—Ōta Yōko, *City of Corpses*

Chapters 5 and 7 of this book read selected fragments by David
Wojnarowicz and Sue Golding, fragments that come from within
the utter destitution of the apocalypse, from within an apocalyptic
destitution that is neither merely a state of being, such as could become simply an object of and for epistemological surveillance, nor
merely the eternality of the "flux." At the same time, they constitute
attempts to think the thought of the historico-social as such, and
hence the essential possibility of the ethico-political, from within
and as the material specificity of that destitution. These texts inscribe the impossibility of their possibility; in this sense, they will
strike many readers as anarcho-terrorist.

Hence, much must be refused here, and that refusal, that negativity, constitutes in large part the work (*travail*) of these fragments;
this labor of refusal and the negative is unavoidable, in the strongest
sense of the term. What is refused here (and, however unavoidable,
it is no simple refusal, a point to which I shall return) is any conception of the sufficiency of the instrumentality of the subject/ob-
ject relation (of a technological rationality, therefore)—construed
as the relation of a knowing subject, constituted in the intuition of
the a priori of space and time, to the objects of the world (and
world as object)—to found the cultural as such, as well as its puta-

tively consequent rationality. What will be thought here, what must
be thought here, is the thought of the surplus, excess, or supplement of that relation—a surplus, an excess, a supplementarity that is
the erotic (as nonrelating relation); it must be emphasized that the
erotic does not simply displace the instrumentality of the subject/
object relation, but exists only in the transgression of that relation.
The fact that the erotic cannot exist except as supplementarity is a
historical necessity.

Consequently, any concept of the sufficiency of the *domus*, the
domestic economy of the technological *and* the ground of cultural
community (as *Heimat*, *ie*, or *habitus*) is refused in the thought of
the city, in the thought of what Paul Hallam has called Sodom.[56]
This thought of the city is the thought of the insufficiency of the
concept of the domus to account for, or even speak to, the radically exorbitant surplus or waste, the *désoeuvrée*, of culture. What is
at issue here is not a matter of marginality, the thought of which
relegates the difference of supplementarity to a simple outside, leaving the domus intact. Rather, the thought of the city is the thought
of a difference residing at what is putatively the heart of the cultural. What is refused here is a concept of cultural community or
"society" or "humanity" as constituted in the intersubjective recognition of an essential similitude; what is thought here is the essential
promiscuity of the nonrelating relation of infinite singularities, the
infinite proliferation of difference. Wojnarowicz and Golding do
not "have dates"; what queerness means here is the impossibility of
a *queer* soap opera; in other words, what is thought here is love and
pleasure rather than desire, an uncommon being-in-common that *is*
the essential impossibility of reducing the social to any humanism.
What is most radical here, of course, is the erotic conjunction of an
essentially unreserved love and pleasure, bypassing the courses of
desire. This is at once the affirmation of a being-in-common (as
queers) and the negation thereof, and the affirmation thereof *in* its
negation—an essentially *perverse* nonpositive affirmation; it is this
nonpositive affirmation of our impossible commonality (and community in its *perversity*) that is here designated by the term "queer."

Concomitantly, there is equally a refusal here of any concept of politics as the struggle for hegemony and the liberal adjudication of differing private interests and of power relations within the public sphere, a liberalism that assumes that the political as such is always a present possibility. In Wojnarowicz and Golding, there is a thought of politicality, of the political as such, which is to say of the ethicopolitical, in a time in which the possibility for the political has become occluded in its representation, and in its occlusion foreclosed. Here politicality is affirmed as the radical unjustifiability of what is in its infinite, anonymous, destitute singularity. What is affirmed as the surplus or supplement of politics is the ethico-political; but it is affirmed as the nonpositive affirmation of force (the radical unjustifiability of being) and the absolute contingency of the political relation altogether: this affirmation constitutes a *sovereign perversity*.

This sovereign perversity of the ethico-political as such is a matter of a writing, an Imaginary, that is also always something other than representation. This is a witnessing or testimony, as in Ōta and Takenishi, to the unrepresentability of historicity within any historiographical Imaginary; but it is at the same time testimony to the fact that *there is* history, testimony to the exigency that the existential poses and to the exigency that *is* the existential, testimony to the "il y a" or "Es gibt" of historicity. This testimony, which is the supplement of representation, constitutes no work (*oeuvre*); it is a radically désoeuvrée writing. Such a labor is without result, although it is not without its effects; it results in no culture, no *Bildung*, and constructs no community, for what is communicated is the failure of communication, a failure which is that limit of communication which can only be encountered by means of communication. This writing is thus no mere "response" to the exigency of the existential; it does not merely record the "experience" of the limit before the surveillance of the epistemological Gaze. Rather, this writing *is* itself the experience of the limit. Both Wojnarowicz and Golding testify to the erotic, the historico-social, the ethico-political, and their conjunction as limit-experience in a writing that is itself the experience of the limit, a "sovereign" writing, a *perverse* writing, an erotics of thought, a *political* writing, undertaken in the interest of disclosing the political. These fragments thus constitute—if anything—a politics of inconsolable perversity.

It should be emphasized yet again that these movements, these migrations, these metamorphoses, from the domus to the city, from the technological to the erotic, from a humanist *socius* to the social, from the politics of liberalism to the ethico-political, from representation to a sovereign perverse writing, are not optional; these movements are not merely possible transactions in a theoretico-philosophical agora. Only in part are they interventions in the "conflict of interpretations"; moreover, they are interventions only insofar as they call into question the very possibility of interpretation. It is not possible to abstain from the historicity of that force of outside that *is* the exigency of the existential. It should also be yet again emphasized that these fragments anticipate no utopia, they do not constitute a simple rejection or negation of that which they do in fact reject or negate; it is only in their apocalyptic and destitute rejection of the future that they open the possibility of a futurity that, as Gramsci argued, will not be ours to know. What follows is an attempt, in tracing what I conceive to be the most radical peripeteia of these fragments, to begin to think what is unavoidable for thought in this interminable time of AIDS.

In tracing the peripeteia of these fragments I am undoubtedly tracing and retracing the narrative figure, the fable, of a logic—from the impossible ground of a historicity (as the apocalyptic, destitute finitude of being) to the erotic, to a consideration of socialty, the ethico-political, and, finally, of writing. But it should of course be kept in mind that this narrative is nothing more—and nothing less—than a figure, neither more nor less than a fable. What I read to be written in Wojnarowicz and Golding, no less than in Takenishi and Ōta, is the precedence of a logic, a figure, perhaps even a schema, that is not the expression of an immanence, but of a thinking that is the thought of the limits of the thinkable—which can never be a story.

The radical historicity that limns the figure of this logic, this logical fable, is instituted, then, in Wojnarowicz in a double articulation:

I found that, after witnessing Peter Hujar's death on November 26, 1987, and after my recent diagnosis, I tend to dismantle and discard any and all kinds of spiritual and psychic and physical words or concepts designed to make sense of the external world or designed to give momentary comfort. . . . I suddenly resist comfort, from myself and especially from others. There is something I want to see clearly, something I want to witness in its raw state. And this need comes from my sense of mortality. . . . I'm a prisoner of language that doesn't have a letter or a sign or gesture that approximates what I'm sensing.⁵⁷

A double articulation: the death of the singular other (Peter Hujar) and the diagnosis, which is perhaps no mere memento mori. What is in any case at stake in this double articulation is the sense (intuition?) that there is that (death, apocalyptic destitution, finitude) which is radically unsignifiable, which can never become signification but is nevertheless the ground of *signifiance* as the possibility for, and the process of bringing into being, any signification whatsoever. And this "that which" is occluded by signification, sense, intelligibility. This *occlusion* is what Wojnarowicz continually refers to as the "preinvented world," which is in fact the forgetting of the radical finitude—or destitution—of being. Here in Wojnarowicz, then, is no mere impossibility of the work of mourning, the consolations of intelligibility, but the necessary *refusal* of every transcendence, an impossible desire to engage the apocalyptic as "something I want to see clearly, something I want to witness in its raw state." I shall return to these themes.

In any event, what is at stake in the first instance, in the death of the singular other, is a certain punctuation: Peter Hujar, November 1987 (to which we must now add: David Wojnarowicz, August 1992), the name and the date, now forever indivisible, indicating the originary separation ("death") that is the condition of possibility for historical consciousness. "Peter Hujar" henceforth will name not only the instance of an intersubjective recognition, but also both the impossibility and surplus of that recognition. "Peter Hujar" will be both name and anonym. In the wake of the death of Peter Hujar, a narrative voice, which I shall very problematically name David Wojnarowicz, records the attempt to bring the death of Peter Hujar

to signification—for example, "to make a film that records the rituals in an attempt to give grief form" (*CK*, 100). As part of this attempt, Wojnarowicz visits Hujar's grave; "suspending all disbelief"
(*CK*, 101), he interpellates his friend who, in the presence of his
absence (for Wojnarowicz is convinced Hujar witnesses the interpellation), the failure of his response, gives the lie to the intersubjective relation, but who in the failure to respond recalls to Wojnarowicz the possibility of an intersubjective relation:

> And his death is now as if it's printed on celluloid on the backs of
> my eyes. [The form of a certain formlessness, therefore.] That last
> day . . . there was some point when I was sitting at the far corner of
> the bed in a chair thinking about leaving when I looked toward his
> face and his eyes moved slightly and I put two fingers up like rabbit
> ears behind the back of my head, a gesture, a high sign we had that
> we'd discreetly give when we bumped into each other at a crowded
> gathering in the past. I flashed him the sign and then turned away
> embarrassed and moments later Ethyl said, "David . . . look at Peter."
> We all turned to the bed and his body was completely still; and then
> there was a very strong and slow intake of breath and then stillness
> and then one more intake of breath and he was gone. (*CK*, 102)

This sign, this punctuation, whatever "message" it may in fact have
communicated (which must remain forever undecidable and inde-
cipherable), communicated at least the possibility of communication, the recognition of an other as the possibility for language,
communication, and sociality. But this sign, this punctuation, also, of
course, signals what will henceforth be the impossibility of language,
communication, and sociality. Thus that punctuality (the "just then"
that interrupts every phenomenological temporality) that *is* "Peter
Hujar; November 26, 1987," registers at once the possibility and
impossibility of recognition, language, and sociality. It is the death of
an other that discloses the apocalyptic destitution of being, beyond
every consolation of intelligibility. Perhaps it is this, the untenable
ground of *signifiance*, that Wojnarowicz wanted to witness "in its
raw state."

The unsignifiable, the historicity that is both the ground of *signifiance* and its impossibility, is at the same time also articulated in

Wojnarowicz in terms of the "diagnosis" (no need any more to ask *what* is being diagnosed), the certification of his mortality and fini-tude. Succinctly: "THERE IS SOMETHING IN MY BLOOD AND IT S TRYING TO FUCKING KILL ME."[58] Certainly, a number of themes that are all too disastrously familiar to us from thousands of testimonies to the impact of "the diagnosis" surface here—the theme of the alien within and the consequent problematization of the very categories of "inside" and "outside"; or the establishment of "the diagnosis" as the barrier that henceforth divides a pre-test "before" (often re-called in nostalgia) from the horrors of an unavoidable ever-after or forever-more, for example.[59] What I think bears emphasis here, in the double articulation or punctuation of historicity, is the uncertain punctuality by which the diagnosis guarantees a certain impossibil-ity of hermeneutic redemption for the subject. What Wojnarowicz is refusing are the consolations of a certain prolepsis, the transcen-dence of the future anterior; what Wojnarowicz is insisting upon, in the refusal of a proleptic work of mourning, is the recognition of the absolute destitution of the material body, which can only be situated in the here and now of an essentially ungraspable present. Thus, in an essay entitled "Postcards from America," and aptly sub-titled "X Rays from Hell" (*CK*, 111–23), Wojnarowicz situates the infected body as the locus of an inescapable "intense claustrophobic feeling of fucking doom" (*CK*, 112). Elsewhere, at the bedside of a dying friend (Peter Hujar?), he wrote, "at the moment I'm a six-teen-foot-tall five-hundred-and-forty-eight-pound man inside this six-foot body and all I can feel is the pressure all I can feel is the pressure and the need for release" (*CK*, 83).

Before "the diagnosis" the site of an erotic encounter with al-terity, the material body is henceforth also, and increasingly, in its es-sential claustrophobia and in its pain, the very impossibility of flight, avoidance, movement. As Jacques Lacan argues, the claustrophobia that is pain constitutes the limit that is its existentiality, its historic-ity; thus, "we should perhaps conceive of pain as a field which, in the realm of existence, opens precisely onto that limit where a living being has no possibility of escape."[60] The diagnosis is therefore not merely the guarantee of a telos, destiny, or fate, that which lies in wait for all of us "out there," but is equally the guarantee that that death, that historicity, that finitude is here and now: this moment *is* the moment of death. In other words, to live in the world after the diagnosis, *post iudicium*, is to live in the mode of what Giorgio Agamben, reading Robert Walser, calls the irreparable: "Irreparable means that these things are consigned without remedy to their being-thus, that they are precisely and only their *thus*, . . . but irreparable also means that for them there is literally no shelter possible, that in their being-thus they are absolutely exposed, absolutely abandoned."[61] For Wojnarowicz, the thought of transcendence is a "luxury"; the diagnosis, as the index of existentiality and historicity, introduces the subject to the irreparable, for "each day's dose of medicine, or the intermittent aerosol pentamidine treatments, or the sexy stranger nodding to you on the street corner or across the room at a party, reminds you in a clearer than clear way that at this point in history the virus'[s] activity is forever" (*CK*, 188).

If, in this logical fable I am retracing, the articulation of apocalyptic destitution of being in its existentiality is a kind of phenomenological punctuation—that is, the limit of phenomenological apprehension altogether—this historicity is also, and perhaps essentially for Wojnarowicz, that which is occluded by the "preinvented world"; for, to return to one of the elisions in the quotation that opened this reading of Wojnarowicz,

> [T]here is a relief in having this sense of mortality. At least I won't arrive one day at my eightieth birthday and at the eve of my possible death and only then realize my whole life was supposed to be somewhat a preparation for the event of death and suddenly fill up with rage because instead of preparation all I had was a lifetime of adaption to the preinvented world—do you understand what I'm saying here? . . . I'm trying to lift off the weight of the preinvented world so I can see what's underneath it all. I'm hungry and the preinvented world won't satisfy my hunger. (*CK*, 116–17)

There is a demand here, one constantly reiterated, for an engagement with the radical historicity or finitude of existentiality, which is thereby a demand for an engagement with the very instauration of *significance*, culture, and sociality—a *revolutionary* engagement, therefore—and this cannot be taken merely for a demand for any phenomenological (least of all psychological) authenticity, because this historicity is originarily articulated in relation to the always-already-there of the preinvented world, in relation to the inscriptions of the cultural domus, the inscription of the cultural as such, its structures and representations, and its assumption of a preternatural normativity, which, in occluding historicity, constitute a forgetting, the forgetfulness of being (and thereby foreclose upon the possibility of sociality and politicality altogether).

First and last, when it is a question of going to ground, it is a question of the ground of *signifiance*, the possibility and production of what is called language, of signification, representation, and intelligibility, of the logos as such. It is a question of the limits of any conception of language, representation, and intelligibility that would sustain the assumption that language reduced to its denotative instrumentality might adequately speak the unspeakable, the thought that "the sounds of vessels of blood and muscles contracting the sounds of aging and disintegration" might ever be anything other than "the sound of something made ridiculous with language" (*CK*, 86). In another essay, Wojnarowicz, sluggish and lethargic in a hotel room in Merida, goes to a bullfight, "hoping the sight of blood would shake me up and wake me up to all that which had no words" (*CK*, 257–58). Instrumental rationality reaches its apotheosis, if not its telos, at the "air force museum of the atomic bomb," where the celebratory *representation of* instrumental rationality serves precisely and explicitly to obviate any reflection upon or engagement with that instrumental mastery's effects. Thus, the narrator muses that "if I owned the place I'd hook the constant smell of rotting flesh into the air-conditioning unit and have all the screens filled with speeded-up films of rotting corpses" (*CK*, 37). It is not merely that language is inadequate to the representation of what is in its historicity, in its abject destitution, but that as an accomplished signification, and all the possibilities sustained by an accomplished signification, it *precludes* an engagement with the historicity and *signifiance* that is its condition of possibility, a historicity and *signifiance* that thereby become the surplus of signification and sense. But there is that which, insistently, gives the lie to its occlusion in signification and representation:

> You can't shut out the sights and sounds of death, the people waking up with the diseases of small birds or mammals; the people whose faces are entirely black with cancer eating health salads in the lonely seats of restaurants. Those images hurl themselves from the corners of a fast-paced city and you can't even imagine death properly enough to tell this guy what he's railing against. (*CK,* 67)

Following the death of a "he" (who may or may not be "Peter Hujar"), the narrator of "Being Queer in America" (*CK,* 64–83) walks the streets of the city, a city that exists only in the interstices of the domus, the Heimat, the habitus, a city of an utterly abject destitution, peopled by queers, drug users, sex workers, the detritus of the domus or of what Wojnarowicz calls the "One-Tribe Nation," an interstitial city of corpses (*CK,* 67–68). The narrator is "consumed by the emptiness and void surrounding and lying beneath each and every action I witness of others and myself" (*CK,* 68); that which necessarily escapes every signification, that which is therefore sense-less, is therefore the radical absence of ground of the being-in-common of "others" and "myself." Thus, "each little gesture in the movements of the planets" helps "to continue the slow death of ourselves, the slow motion approach of the unveiling of our order and disorder in its ultimate climax" (*CK,* 68): it is the radical historicity of thought (or of history) that undoes (shall we say *deconstructs?*) the very separation of order and disorder that grounds the cultural as such. The operation or movement of this unveiling of the absence of ground of being has a center that is "octopal in its appendages," which "vibrate stroboscopically," and are therefore visible, "if one could withstand the light," only in an ungraspable fulguration, which can only be apprehended as the trace of an image. So,

> [t]he center is something outside of what we know as visual, more a sensation: a huge fat clockwork of civilizations; the whole onward crush of the world as we know it; all the walking swastikas yap-yapping cartoon video death language; a malfunctioning cannonball filled

with bone and gristle and gearwheels and knives and bullets and an-
imals rotting with skeletal remains and pistons and smokestacks pump-
pumping cinders and lightning and shreds of flesh, spewing language
and motions and shit and entrails in its wake. It's all swirling in every
direction simultaneously so that it's neither going forward nor back-
ward, nor from side to side, embracing stasis beyond the ordinary
sense of stillness one witnesses in death, in a decaying corpse that lasts
millions of years in comparison to the sense of time this thing oper-
ates within. This is the vision I see beneath the tiniest gesture of wip-
ing one's lips after a meal or observing a traffic light. (*CK*, 69)

Thus it is that the gestures constitutive of the cultural as such occlude the apocalyptic destitution of a world of corpses.

There are two "worlds," then, the "World" and the "Other
World," which is the historically overdetermined world of the always-already-there of cultural inscriptions and thereby of the inscription of culture as such, the "preinvented world" (or "Universe
of the Neatly Clipped Lawn"), which is the entire congeries of tattoos, scars, brands, and blazons inscribed on and as the "body," by
which we presume to recognize the body "as such":

First there is the World. Then there is the Other World. The Other
World is where I sometimes lose my footing. In its calendar turnings,
in its preinvented existence. The barrage of twists and turns where I
sometimes get weary trying to keep up with it, minute by minute
adapt: the world of the stoplight, the no-smoking signs, the rental
world, the split-rail fencing shielding hundreds of miles of barren
wilderness from the human step. A place where by virtue of having
been born centuries late one is denied access to earth or space, choice
or movement. The bought-up world; the owned world. The world of
coded sounds: the world of language, the world of lies. The pack-
aged world; the world of speed in metallic motion. The Other World
where I've always felt like an alien. But there's the World where one
adapts and stretches the boundaries of the Other World through keys
of the imagination. But then again, the imagination is encoded with
the invented information of the Other World. One stops before a
light that turns from green to red and one grows centuries old in that
moment. Someone once said that the Other World was run by a different species of humans. It is the distance of stepping back or slow-
ing down that reveals the Other World. It's the dislocation of response

that reveals it for the first time because the Other World gets into one's bloodstream with the invisibility of a lover. It slowly takes the shape of the cells and their growth, internalized until it becomes an extension of the body. Traveling into primitive cultures allows one a sudden and clear view of the Other World; how the invention of the word "nature" disassociates us from the ground we walk on. (*CK*, 87–88)

It is only in what we shall see to be a necessarily violent dislocation or distantiation that the Other World can be objectified as a historical construct; what we take to be its connaturality, which is to say its necessity, its ahistoricity, can be exposed in its essential artifice only in a violence (however Imaginary) that disturbs the assumption that "culture" is a separation *from* "nature." Paradoxically, it is precisely in that assumption that the preinvented world can lay claim to its own connaturality, the necessity of order and the cultural as such.

Certainly, what Wojnarowicz variously calls the Other World, the preinvented world, or the Universe of the Neatly Clipped Lawn is a profoundly alienated and alienating world, the "world" *as* alienation, *as* a profound, perhaps in some aspects originary, inauthenticity. But does that make of the "world," that interstitial World visible only in its traces, a "world" of nonalienation, of authenticity, of a kind of ontological *jouissance*? Yes, perhaps, but with essential qualifications, qualifications that make it impossible to conceive of the "World" as the simple outside of the fundamental regulation or order of the cultural as such, qualifications that essentially problematize any notion that the "World" in Wojnarowicz is simply the impossible "object" of an aesthetic sublime within which self would become orgasm and the "World" an amniotic plenitude:

> Previously, before leaving the city to go someplace else for a long time, the city would suddenly change. It was revealed to me as if I had let go of something that was keeping it hidden. Wonderful things tended to happen or reveal themselves in the days before departure. Life or living seemed quite an amazing spectacle. There was humanity beneath every gesture moving along the sidewalks. It was a sudden vision of the World, a transient position of the body in relation to

the Other World. I came to understand that to give up one's environment was to also give up biography and all the encoded daily
movements: those false reassurances of the railing outside the door.
This was the beginning of a definition of the World for me. A place
that might be described as interior world. The place where movement was comfortable, where boundaries were stretched or obliterated: no walls, borders, language or fear. (*CK*, 108)

To belabor the obvious, perhaps, the World, or a "sudden vision of
the World," only appears in relation (albeit a relation of nonrelation, a departure) to the Other World; the "amazing spectacle" is a
glimpse, not of a new heaven and a new earth, but of a transformation or metamorphosis of the Other World, "a transient position of the body to the Other World"; that which inhabits the
Other World as the transformative possibility of the Other World.
Further, the World appears only *in* and *as* anticipation, in the mode
of a certain limnality, therefore; the World is illuminated only in respect of, and *as*, the disclosure of the transience, impermanence,
historicity of the Other World (and thus seems to approach Heidegger's notion of *alētheia*). In spite of the fact that the World is
imagined in terms of interiority, *what* is anticipated is a becoming-
other, a radical loss of "self": to give up one's "environment"—the
"encoded daily movements," the "false reassurances of the railing
outside the door," which, as we also saw in Ōta, constitute subjectivity as such—is to give up "biography." Thus, the World is not,
in fact, a destination, a destiny, a telos, that which would accomplish a fully constituted and realized subjectivity: the nonalienation
or noninauthenticity of the World is not thereby a presence to self.

    And all of this constitutes an engagement with the exigency of
the existential that is historicity. The passage (in every sense of the
term) continues:

With the appearance of AIDS and the sense of mortality I now find
everything revealing itself to me in this way. The sense that came
about in moments of departure occurs, only now I don't even have to
go anywhere. It is the possibility of departure in a final sense, a sense
called death that is now opening up the gates. Where once I felt
acutely alien, now it's more like an immersion in a body of warm

water and the water that surrounds me is air, is breathing, is life itself. I'm acutely aware of myself alive and witnessing. . . . Time is now compressed. . . . I work quickly now and feel there is no time for bullshit. Cut straight to the heart of the senses and map it out as clearly as tools and growth allow. In better moments I can see my friends—vague transparencies of their faces maybe over my shoulder or superimposed on the surfaces of my eyes—making me more aware of myself, seeing myself from a distance, seeing myself seeing others. I can almost see my own breath, see my internal organs functioning pump pumping. These days I see the edge of mortality. The edge of death and dying is around everything like a warm halo of light sometimes dim sometimes irradiated. I see myself seeing death. (*CK*, 108–9)

If the World thus appears only in the interstices, syncopes, lapses, and discontinuities of the Other World, it does so only as a zero-degree *aisthēsis*, which always evades the aesthetic (including the aesthetic of the sublime) and is nonalienation only insofar as it opens upon, in an "aletheic" mode, the erotic "as such," the social "as such," and hence the possibility for the ethico-political "as such." If the World thus constitutes in some sense the impossible object of an essentially insatiable desire, that desire can "itself" only be disclosed through the courses of pleasure or, in more general terms, the erotic: "Cut straight to the heart of the senses and map it out as clearly as tools and growth allow." A parable, then, for the relation of a radical historicity to the essential domestic regulation of the Other World:

I remembered a friend of mine dying from AIDS, and while he was visiting his family on the coast for the last time, he was seated in the grass during a picnic to which dozens of family members were invited. He looked up from his fried chicken and said, "I just want to die with a big dick in my mouth." (*CK*, 44)

The Erotic

What is at stake in Wojnarowicz when it is the relation of "sex" to an engagement with the radical historicity of being that is at stake? What is at stake when it is the coincidence of "sex" and "death" that is at stake? What is at stake in the intense homoeroticism, not only of his writing, but of many of the visual images he produced, most especially in view of his explicit refusal to differentiate between "pornography" and "erotica" (*CK*, 144)? I want to argue that, at least in terms of the logical fable I am attempting to retrace, "sex" is the passage to, and as passage *is*, the opening onto the erotic. We should not, of course, make the mistake of assuming the identity of what counts as sex and the erotic. Sex is not necessarily eroticizable (consider, for example, the description of what amounts to a rape of the narrator at age fifteen [*MSG*, 15–26]); conversely, erotic relations are not necessarily what count as "sex." At the same time, in no way does the erotic relation necessarily exclude sexual relations of whatever kind (and in fact, Wojnarowicz explicitly privileges sexual relations); and sexual relations always imply at least the possibility of an opening on to the erotic. The erotic, I argue, designates in Wojnarowicz the surplus, excess, or supplement of the subject/object relation, both the *technē* the subject/object relation implies and the rationality within which it is constituted. As surplus or supplement, it is a *transgression of* the subject/object relation and its technological rationality, and it is thus in some sense bound to that relation. But the erotic is not, by virtue of its very supplementarity, subsidiary or secondary with respect to the subject/object relation: the subject/object relation and the erotic are *equiprimordial*. The erotic is thus the privileged mode of nontranscendence, our "access to" nontranscendence, or to a "finite transcendence" (Fynsk) in which it is the existential (what Wojnarowicz calls the "World") that exceeds, transgresses, or transcends the "Other World" or any possible *thought of* the existential; in this sense, the erotic designates the force of the Outside. The erotic therefore opens upon a sociality quite other than the regulated social relations of the preinvented world *in* and *as* it transgresses the boundaries of those relations in their regularity. The erotic is the ground of sociality as such, and thereby the possibility for the political as such.

It is, in Wojnarowicz, first of all a matter of a passage, which is always, as we have seen, a departure, a detour, a *détournement*, and thereby of a queer perversity: "I hate highways but love speeding and I can only think of men's bodies" (*MSG*, 9), as one of Wojnarowicz's narrators maintains, as he moves "into the drift and sway" of a series of homoerotic encounters. Indeed, "[d]riving a machine through the days and nights of the empty and pressurized landscape eroticizes the whole world flitting in through the twin apertures of the eyes" (*CK*, 26). Elsewhere in the same essay, but again driving, the narrator will say, "I'm getting closer to the coast and realize how much I hate arriving at a destination. Transition is always a relief. Destination means death to me. If I could figure out a way to remain forever in transition, in the disconnected and unfamiliar, I could remain in a state of perpetual freedom" (*CK*, 62). This celebration of perpetual movement can be read, of course, as the valorization of a Bergsonian pure duration or of an unconstrained motility and of the flux; but it is inflected, perhaps deflected, by the fact that it is always a departure, a separation, a secession *from* the preinvented Other World, in respect of which this flight is always a turning, always necessarily perverse, the *ekstasis* that is the very cutting edge of metamorphosis—or of revolution. This movement describes a curve (in which every point is determinative rather than determined), obliterated in and as its very inscription, an itinerary that leaves no traces. What seduces Wojnarowicz here, as it were, is the perverse edge or bite of liminality, the queer turn.

Concomitantly, what will also be at stake in the erotic for Wojnarowicz will be the emergence, or rather the eruption, of the figural, the ungraspable moment in which form erupts, the very *signifiance* of the Imaginary. What fascinates Wojnarowicz are the lines, boundaries, and limits that both separate and connect, are neither inside nor outside, but both inside and outside, at which the form they would delineate both appears and disappears: the line, the boundary, the limit as lamellae. What emerges here is therefore not a Euclidean geometry of forms and hence of significations, but a topology of *signifiance*. Thus, what draws Wojnarowicz's attention, in an essay entitled "Losing the Form in Darkness" (*CK*, 9–23), is a certain *turning*, "the simple sense of turning slowly, feeling the breath of another body in a quiet room, the stillness shattered by the scraping of a fingernail against a collar line. Turning is the motion that disrupts the vision. . . . It is the motion that sets into trembling the subtle water movements of shadows, like lines following the disappearance of a man beneath the surface of an abandoned lake" (*CK*, 10). Or the "discrete pleasures" (which will never coalesce in the unity of desire) of the line: "Old images race back and forth and I'm gathering a heat in the depths of my belly from them: flashes of a curve of arm, back, the lines of a neck glimpsed among the crowds in the train stations, one that you could write whole poems to" (*CK*, 12). Or it will be a temporal lamella, the indeterminate punctuality of the "just when" that links day to night, which is neither day nor night, which is both day and night, the disjunct simultaneity of day and night, which will be essentially, in its nonessentiality, erotic: "When he lifted away from my chest I saw his eyes, the irises the color of dark chips of stone, something like the sky at dusk after a clear hot summer day, when the ships are folding down into the distance and jet exhaust trails are uttered from the lips of strangers" (*CK*, 15–16; 18). Indeed, dusk was one of Wojnarowicz's "favorite times of day," he asserted in an interview with Barry Blinderman.[62] Hermaphroditism (*CK*, 18) and the interval between sleeping and waking (*CK*, 24, 173) disclose the erotic for him as well; above all, it is the horizon where sky meets the ocean that is the site of the finite transcendence that is nontranscendence. "[I]f you see nothing," he advises a friend who is on the verge of death, suspended in the disjunct simultaneity of life and death, "then try to imagine that one period of calm in the midst of that sky just where it reaches the ocean. That one place I've always seen as a point of time and space where everything is possible, where I could dream myself anywhere in any position and I said move into that, become that, merge with it. Death" (*CK*, 82).

If such lamellae are in themselves the *ekstases* of metamorphosis, of a becoming-other, the punctuality or "just then" of ecstasy, then the "fracture of orgasm" (*CK*, 57), and jouissance will itself be a topological lamella:

I lay in a hotel room one night after selling my body to a customer who had gone back home to his wife and kids, and I wished I'd had a motorcycle and that I was in a faraway landscape, maybe someplace out west. I saw myself riding this machine faster and faster and faster toward the edge of a cliff until I hit the right speed that would take me off the cliff in a arcing motion. At that instant when my body and the machine cleared the edge of the cliff and hit the point in the sky where I was neither rising nor falling—somewhere in there: once my body and the motorcycle hit a point in the light and wind and loss of gravity, in that exact moment, I would suddenly disappear, and the motorcycle would continue the downward arc of gravity and explode into flames somewhere among the rocks at the bottom of the cliff. And it is in that sense of void—that marriage of body-machine and space—where one should most desire a continuance of life, that I most wish to disappear. I realized that the image of the point of marriage between body-vehicle and space was similar to the beginning of orgasm. (*CK*, 41)

To underscore the obvious, it is not the accomplishment of a putative satisfaction that is of interest here, but the very movement of pleasure, the transgression of a limit, the being at the limit, the ungraspable limit-situation *itself* that is essentially erotic, and is perhaps as close as it is possible to come to the "essence" of the erotic. If the erotic as such is characterized as a limit-situation, the limit-situation that is the finite transcendence of the nontranscendence of the existential—the Real—then it is there that the a priori intuitions of space and time, the possibility for subjectivity-as-synthesis (and for synthetic judgments), are called into radical question. The *essentially* discrete pleasures of the erotic can never be brought together into the synthetic unity of a subject's erotobiography; the erotic for Wojnarowicz is *essentially* fragmentary, dispersed, a relation of nonrelation, a disjunct simultaneity, always evading signification and meaning, in fine: nontranscendent. Bodies, "pieces of anatomy" (*CK*, 25), lines, pleasures, vision, syntagmas, all bespeak the finite transcendence of the erotic in their originary and equiprimordial punctuality or fragmentation (a fragmentation that is thereby not the misfortune of a dismemberment that befalls the body, the line, the image, the syntagma):

Turning the bend in the highway suddenly reveals, a quarter mile away, a highway crew standing in a jumble of broken earth and enormous machines. In that instance I see the browned flesh of a shirtless man in shorts; I see the bare arms and ribs of a man buried in the shadows of a tractor's cab; I see the bent-over back of a man swinging a pickax with all his might; I see the pale white underarm with the accompanying dark spot of wet hair belonging to a guy up in a cherry picker among the telephone wires and I feel the fist of tension rising through my solar plexus beneath my t-shirt and the sensation grows upward, spreading like some strange fever in my chest, catching only at the throat where small pockets of sound are contained. In a moment the vehicle I'm steering passes by the scene and I'm left populating the dry plains, the buttes and the cloudless sky with the touch and taste of flesh. I fill the gullies with small but heated fictions.

There is really no difference between memory and sight, fantasy and actual vision. (*CK*, 26)

As with the erotic "pieces of anatomy" that refuse to coalesce into a unitary "body," so too vision itself is "made up of millions of tiny stills as in transparencies" (*CK*, 53); thus, discussing his photography, Wojnarowicz records that "photographs are like words and I generally will place many photographs together or print them one inside the other in order to construct a free-floating sentence that speaks about the world I witness" (*CK*, 144). For example, undoubtedly:

I hate highways but love speeding and I can only think of men's bodies and the drift and sway of my own if sex was a dance I'd do a crawl for that body I saw this afternoon the guy stepping out from the cab of his truck in the parking lot of the bus stop he looked kinda canadian and in a sexy collared shirt and tight faded jeans and thick leather belt and boots and a crease in the front of his pants that let his dick rest lazy and calm and forearms I'd want under my tongue and after the turn on the bridge when I'd swung back going north stopped at a rest stop and a truck pulled in I walked past it a little later and a ruby red light flicked on and a silhouette of a man in worker's pants stepped out swinging from the bar next to the outside rear view mirror and walked past me in a blaze of car lights and entered the bathroom. (*MSG*, 9–12)

In the erotic, *significance* constitutes a movement that at once accomplishes signification and withdraws or secedes from signification and from the signification that is the syntagma, into an originary fragmentation that cannot be construed as the degeneration or dissolution of an always already established signified. The image of the "body" in its integral unity is always already also the *corps morcelé*; the erotic movement of *significance* is at once the accomplishment of sense and its excess, the fragmentation and proliferation of sensuous non-sense, the operation or work (*travail*) that simultaneously accomplishes a work (*oeuvre*) and its unworking (*désoeuvrée*).

That nontranscendence or finite transcendence, the relation of a nonrelation to the Real or existentiality, which "is" the erotic, appears, as it were, only in and as the syncopes of the transgression of the order of the preinvented Other World, which in fact occludes the erotic. The erotic, therefore, cannot be a "state of being," but is only disclosed as the ekstasis that is the cutting edge, the bite, of metamorphosis, the very transitivity of be-ing. Thus far, for the purposes of this logical fable that I am attempting to retrace, I have isolated (an isolation that is entirely fictive) four aspects or "moments" of the essentially ungraspable, unpossessable, erotic.

1. The erotic erupts in and as that which precipitates the movement of a departure, a withdrawal, a secession without destination—as death.

2. The erotic is always a turning, a détournement, a perversity, a queering of an itinerary: the erotic is not for such men as go straight to the point. The erotic itinerary is always the edge of a curve; more, a topology: neither obverse nor reverse, both obverse and reverse, a lamella.

3. The erotic is the punctuality of a temporal-corporeal ekstasis, the precipitating of orgasm. In the erotic, one always comes on time, which is neither the arrival at the destination of a satisfaction nor the recovery of an equilibrium. Rather, the erotic resides in the radical disequilibrium of the strange.

4. The erotic is the very movement of *significance*, the disjunct simultaneity of the achievement of sense and the fragmentation and proliferation of a sensuous non-sense.

It would necessarily follow that in the erotic everything taken to constitute, however informally, the conditions of possibility for a phenomenological auto-affectivity or "sense of self" is called into radical question. The erotic "as such" is a radical loss of self. But it is only from the perspective of the always-already-there of the preinvented Other World that the erotic can be conceived as loss or disintegration, as if the erotic were merely a contingency that befalls the fully constituted self-presence of a phenomenological subject. Contingent the erotic most certainly is, but it is not thereby a phenomenological or psychological misfortune. Rather, the erotic must be thought as a nonintegration rigorously equiprimordial with the putative integrity that is taken to be the self. *Close to the Knives* is undoubtedly, as the subtitle announces, a "journal of disintegration" in the sense of a mortal dissolution; but it is *also* the journal of the radical nonintegration of the erotic. This nonintegration necessarily constitutes a "loss of self" from the perspective of the constituted subjects we always already are.

But Wojnarowicz conceives this erotic "loss" as a liberating movement, which never coalesces into a state of being that would bear the name of liberation or freedom. Encountering a stranger parked by the river, the narrator enters an abandoned structure:

> I lean toward him, pushing him against the wall, lifting my pale hands up beneath his sweater, finding the edge of his tight t-shirt and peeling it upward. I placed my palms against the hard curve of his abdomen, his chest rolling slightly in pleasure. . . . He is sucking and chewing on my neck, pulling my body into his, and over the curve of his shoulder, sunlight is burning through a window emptied of glass. The frame still contains a rusted screen that reduces shapes and colors into tiny dots like a film directed by Seurat. . . . I lean down and find the neckline of his sweater and draw it back and away from the nape of his neck which I gently probe with my tongue. In loving him, I saw a cigarette between the fingers of a hand, smoke blowing backwards into the room, and sputtering planes diving low through the clouds. In loving him, I saw men encouraging each other to lay down their arms. In loving him, I saw small-town laborers creating excavations that other men spend their lives trying to fill. In loving him, I saw moving films of stone buildings; I saw a hand in prison dragging

snow in from the sill. In loving him I saw great houses being erected that would soon slide into the waiting and stirring seas. I saw him freeing me from the silences of the interior life. (*CK*, 16–17)

That this passage, in its staging of an erotic sexual encounter, recapitulates many of the thematics of the erotic is readily apparent. What perhaps demands closer attention is that it is "in loving him" that "I saw him freeing me from the silences of the interior life." The erotic relation, the relation that is the relation of nonrelation, is the passage from a monadic interiority to the radical nonintegration of alterity. Undoubtedly, in this sexual encounter, one is simultaneously subject and object for the other, and thereby for himself; the subject/object relation is not transcended in the sense of achieving an undifferentiated union, or therefore in the sense of the accomplishment of a mystical reunion with the Other. At the same time, which means equiprimordially, this erotic relation cannot be reduced to a subject/object relation or mere intersubjectivity, because this relation is not constituted in the recognition of the essential similitude of psychological subjects. Indeed, the eroticism of the encounter depends, essentially, upon the status, perhaps not yet a category, of the stranger. In fact, the physical description of the *stranger*, who *must* remain nameless, is not unlike the description of a fetish:

> He had a tough face. It was square-jawed and barely shaven. Close-cropped hair wiry and black, handsome like some face in old boxer photographs, a cross between an aging boxer and Mayakovsky. He had a nose that might have once been broken in some dark avenue barroom in a distant city invented by some horny young kid. There was a wealth of images in that jawline, slight tension to it and curving down toward a hungry-looking mouth. (*CK*, 14–15)

What is at stake in this description of the stranger-as-fetish is, as with any fetish (which signifies nothing except the erotic altogether: it says only "eroticism"), a singularity that is not the expression of an essence. In his singularity, the stranger exceeds any possible predicate, every subsumption; but because there can therefore be no relation between singularities, the relation between stranger and narrator is, in fact, a nonrelation, the relation that *is* nonrelation. This relation of nonrelation, this singularity, is therefore a nondialectical passage to, and *as*, a radical alterity, and can only be marked as the excess, surplus, or supplement of any possible relation.

Undoubtedly, there is an affirmation here, one of innumerable affirmations of the erotic in the wake of the AIDS pandemic. It is well known, of course, that in the United States in the early 1980's, with the appearance of AIDS and some knowledge of its epidemiology and etiology, there was a more or less widespread reaction against what was regarded as "irresponsible" gay male "behavior," a reaction many saw as foreclosure of many of the sexual and erotic possibilities that had been affirmed by gay liberation movements of the previous decade. This reaction took institutional form in various measures and pronouncements from government at all levels, in the closing of bath houses and other venues of sexual congress catering to gay men, in increased police surveillance of tearooms, in much of the discourse on "safer sex" (which still claims the moral high ground), and in what were perceived to be the moralistic pronouncements of some gay men themselves (Randy Shilts and Larry Kramer, for example). Partly in reaction to this recidivist moralism, a variety of new voices became audible that denounced it in no uncertain terms. I think, for example, of work by Douglas Crimp, Simon Watney, Leo Bersani, Frank Browning, Marlon Riggs, Gary Indiana, David B. Feinberg, Samuel R. Delany; of safer sex "pornography," whether produced with explicit pedagogical intent or not; of the sexual practices of lesbians and gays ourselves (such as j.o. clubs, phone sex, SM practices, a return to the pleasures of cruising, the public inscriptions of Boy with Arms Akimbo ["sex is just sex"], etc.)—and I think, of course, of the work of David Wojnarowicz, which quite explicitly belongs to the reaffirmation of an equally explicit sexual erotics.[63] As much of this work and many of these practices maintain, this reaffirmation is neither merely the reaffirmation of a sexual libertarianism, nor simply the resurgence of a discourse on the liberative revolutionary possibilities of sexuality altogether, as in Herbert Marcuse or Guy Hocquenghem.[64] These reaffirmations may indeed be central to some of what is going on, certainly, but one can also say that, whether explicitly or not, there has also been in these texts and in these practices an increasing attention to what is at stake when it is the erotic that is at stake in "sex." What is at stake when it is the erotic that is at stake is a radical sociality that is at once the condition of possibility for social being and the excess or surplus of any hypostatized objectification denominated "society." Thereby, what is also at stake is the (impossible) ground of the ethico-political.

The Social

So: it is "in *loving* him" that the work (*travail*) and works (*oeuvre*) that institute the cultural as such are disclosed; it is "in *loving* him" that "I saw him freeing me from the silences of the interior life." It is "in *loving* him" that the radical contingency of sociality as such is revealed. To think the contingent encounter of anonymous sexual nomads (who are always on the point of departure) to be an act of loving is to think not only against the denunciation of a promiscuity (a promiscuity that is held to be the very impossibility of love), but also and thereby against hegemonic conceptions of the ground of social being and of "society." To think the erotic encounter with the stranger to be a loving encounter is to think love as the outside of intersubjective recognition, the excess of every psychodrama; something other than a monadic nomadism, the nomadism of every bar's Marlboro men, is at stake here. To rewrite the inscriptions of Boy with Arms Akimbo, it is precisely because "sex is . . . just sex" that sex is never "just sex."

First, the promiscuity of the encounters of sexual nomads, those who always already shall have been on the point of departure, is to think the sexual encounter in view of the relation of nonrelation to the historicity (death, departure) of the other. It makes no difference, really, whether this promiscuous encounter lasts five minutes or fifty years; duration is in fact irrelevant. The promiscuity of the sexual nomad therefore enacts the acknowledgment of the historicity or finitude that is the singularity of any other. The love of this relation of nonrelation constitutes a social bond only in view of that bond's fragility and impermanence, only as an effect of that fragility and impermanence. The social bond must be reinvented, or in fact invented as repetition, at every moment. It is essential to this loving, this loyalty, that it be without guarantee; the sociality of the erotic (and it is this that thereby constitutes the eroticism of the erotic, the turn-on) is grounded in the nothingness that at all points threatens it, in its nonnecessity, its essential insecurity.

Second, because the mode of the promiscuous is that of a contingent historicity, of a nonnecessity, and must thereby (re-)invent the very possibility of sociality at every moment, erotic sociality necessarily implies an essential nonmastery, a noninstrumental usage of the body and of language. Because "the body" in its materiality can be situated nowhere but in the nonpresence of a present, and because this loving is not an affect belonging to a psychological subject but is the relation of nonrelation to the material body of the stranger, the erotic promiscuity of this relation of nonrelation must always figure as the excess, surplus, or supplement of an instrumental subject/object relation (which does not thereby simply disappear). This implies, as we have seen, and as we shall see again in Sue Golding on "Sexual Manners," that the sexual nomad repeatedly returns to the inaugural moment of *signifiance*, at once the achievement and the nonachievement of signification. The rule is a rule only in the act of inscribing the rule; it is not that anything goes, but that regulation is never prior; and it is in this nonpriority, this ungivenness, however Imaginary, of the logos that "the signification of a limitless love [can] emerge, because it is outside the limits of the law, where alone it may live."[65]

Third, this relation of nonrelation to the stranger, this promiscuity of the sexual nomad, this loving, is constituted as an essential nonreserve: "He was whispering behind my closed eyelids. Time had lost its strobic beat and all structures of movement and sensation and taste and sight and sound became fragmented, shifting around like particles in lakewater. I love getting lost like this" (*CK*, 54). This loving, this love, is therefore, as Lacan says somewhere, a "psychological disaster," for in the anonymous singularity of an absolute promiscuity (which is a nonmonogamy even if enacted in the passion of only one other) there is that which transgresses the essential reserve, or "armor," that is the ego. Something more, something other than a mere libidinal cathexis (at least in its normative psychoanalytical constructions), this loving is an existential, rather than psychological, "loss of self," a ruination, a loving *à corps perdu*. There is nothing here, therefore, of the soap opera; these encounters are not "dates." The erotics of the sexual nomad never constitute a psychodrama, and can never become the object of and for a psychology. In putting my "body" in its unobjectifiable materiality at the disposition of the stranger, I affirm what any psychology can conceive only as the ruin or loss of the "self"; and it is precisely this nonreserve, this loving, in its "nondiscrimination," in its nonidentity, that any politics grounded in the notion of identity or the adjudication of "private" interests cannot tolerate. The ego and the identity politics that it implies, constitute the occlusion, and thereby the foreclosure, of the ethico-political: only the essential nonreserve of this promiscuous sociality can open upon the ethico-political. I shall return to this.

Fourth, this sociality is constituted (albeit in a radical contingency) in a no less radical heterogeneity. Promiscuity is frequently thought to be indiscriminate in the sense of an inattention to the punctuality of singularities. Rather, the heterogenous sociality of this erotic nomadism might be thought as what Giorgio Agamben has thought as the "whatever" (*qualunque*): "The Whatever in question here relates to singularity not in its indifference with respect to a common property . . . but only in its being *such as it is.* . . . Love is never directed toward this or that property of the loved one, . . . but neither does it neglect the properties in favor of an insipid generality (universal love): The lover wants the loved one *with all of its predicates*, its being such as it is."[66] In other words, the radical heterogeneity of the social is an encounter, not with the prepredicative other, but with the postpredicative other, "such as it is," at that point at which predication exhausts itself in an infinite congestion of the proper. Yet the mode of being-with for promiscuous sexual nomads is an infinite substitutability, beyond (as transgression and surplus of) every intersubjective relation. The place of this being-with is "Badaliya," the place of an "irrevocable hospitality": "The destruction of the wall dividing [the Talmud's] Eden from Gehenna is thus the secret intention that animates Badaliya. In this community there is no place that is not vicarious, and Eden and Gehenna are only the names of this reciprocal substitution. Against the hypocritical fiction of the unsubstitutability of the individual, which in our culture only serves to guarantee its universal representability, Badaliya presents an unconditioned substitutability, without either representation or possible description—an absolutely unrepresentable community"; "love" is thus "the experience of taking-place in a whatever singularity."[67] The heterogeneity of the social in the infinite punctuality of its attention to singularities "such as they are" is thus not merely a congeries of discrete interests or identities, nor yet is it a universalizing inclusion (which would make of it a mere liberalism); rather, it is a radical nonexclusion. It is not a matter of fucking everything in sight, but rather the insight that there is nothing in principle that is not fuckable.

So the thought of the social, disclosed in the promiscuity of the sexual nomad (and it is important to remember we are trying to image a figure, rather than describe a sociological phenomenon: we are trying to think what is at stake in that being-with which is the condition of possibility of any sociology's object), is the thought of a radical contingency (historicity), the thought of an erotic usage of body and language (the movement of *signifiance*), the thought of an essential nonreserve, the thought of the heterogeneity of the whatever. All of this is what is at stake in the sociality of the sexual nomad in Wojnarowicz, and it is, as Agamben has seen, strictly speaking unrepresentable; it is not an object to which one can point and say that *that* is the social. Sociality is therefore strictly speaking untenable, and it is this very untenability that is affirmed in Wojnarowicz. But it cannot be affirmed as if it existed as some merely alternative state of being, as "liberation" or "freedom," for example. This untenability of being-with can only be affirmed, in a nonpositive affirmation, as that which is occluded and foreclosed by a certain politics, a certain thought of the political; it can only be affirmed in the affirmation of what is excluded by the logic of what

Wojnarowicz calls the "One-Tribe Nation," a logic according to which the sociality that would be its ground can only be constituted in the recognition of an ultimately preternatural similitude, and that must therefore more or less violently expel, as waste, as the abject, that which is—those who are—heterogeneous. The sameness of the community of the One-Tribe nation is inclusive only insofar as it excludes. This is a well-known logic indeed: "we" can form a community of the "we" only in excluding "that" which "we" are *not*. Thus, as Wojnarowicz quotes Sylvère Lotringer, "Our society desperately needs monsters to reclaim its own moral virginity" (*CK*, 192); a "fear of diversity" (*CK*, 154), a radical heterophobia, is the condition of possibility for the one-tribe nation. In Agamben's other, somewhat more formal, terms:

> What the State cannot tolerate in any way, however, is that the singularities form a community without affirming an identity, that humans co-belong without any representable condition of belonging (even in the form a simple presupposition). The State, as Alain Badiou has shown, is not founded on a social bond, of which it would be the expression , but rather on the dissolution, the unbinding it prohibits. For the State, therefore, what is important is never the singularity as such, but only its inclusion in some identity, whatever identity (but the possibility of the *whatever* itself being taken up without an identity is a threat the State cannot come to terms with).[68]

Which means, it would seem, that the thought of the social, in its historicity, in its noninstrumentality, in its nonreserve and in its heterogeneity, must always be thought from within a power relation; and insofar as this thought of the social *is* thought, this thinking the thought of the social must itself be thought as a power relation, at the same time as it is the thought of something other than a power relation. The thought of the social can never be reduced merely to the thought of a negative resistance to the existing order; neither, however, can it ever be thought without the thought of a negative resistance to the existing order. Thus, "[t]o make the *private* into something *public* is an action that has terrific repercussions in the preinvented world" (*CK*, 121). What is at stake here is not merely that "the personal is the political," but that the sociality that is occluded and thereby foreclosed is occluded precisely in the distinction, unthinkable according to any thought of the erotic, between public and private; the "public" expression of that which has been relegated to the invisibility and silence of the "private" therefore calls into radical question the very distinction between public and private. To continue:

> The government has the job of maintaining the day-to-day illusion of the ONE-TRIBE NATION. Each public disclosure of a private reality becomes something of a magnet that can attract others with a similar frame of reference; thus each public disclosure of a fragment of private reality serves as a dismantling tool against the illusion of ONE-TRIBE NATION; it lifts the curtains for a brief peek and reveals the probable existence of literally millions of tribes. The term "general public" disintegrates. What happens next is the possibility of an X-ray of Civilization, an examination of its foundations. (*CK*, 121)

The thematics I have been at pains to develop could not be clearer: the disclosure, however fragmentary and however fleeting, of the social in its essential heterogeneity, in its infinite proliferation of difference, makes the very foundations of the logos—"Civilization"—tremble (or indeed calls into question the very possibility of founding the logos). And this calling into question or solicitation takes a very specific form, that of the political funeral, which was to become in fact one of the practices of ACT UP (and that was an acting upon Wojnarowicz's suggestion, as Jack Ben-Levi has shown in an important essay on Wojnarowicz):[69] "To turn our private grief for the loss of friends, family, lovers *and strangers* into something public would serve as another powerful dismantling tool. . . . One of the first steps in making the private grief public is the ritual of memorials. I have loved the way memorials take the absence of a human being and make them somehow physical with the use of sound" (*CK*, 121; emphasis added).

The rite or ritual of the funeral, a constitutive element of the work of mourning, which is necessarily unaccomplished in Takenishi and Ōta, becomes, in Wojnarowicz, the mark of the existential refusal, the impossibility, of undertaking the historicization of which the funerary ritual is presumptively the instauration; the funeral becomes that which marks the radical destitution or nontranscendence of being. The political funeral becomes the essential perversity that renders any aspiration to redemption or consolation unthinkable; in the political funeral we find a movement toward a politics of inconsolable perversity:

> There is a tendency for people affected by this epidemic to police each other or prescribe what the most important gestures would be for dealing with this experience of loss. I resent that. At the same time, I worry that friends will slowly become professional pallbearers, waiting for each death, of their lovers, friends and neighbors, and polishing their funeral speeches; perfecting their rituals of death rather than a relatively simple ritual of life such as screaming in the streets. I worry because of the urgency of the situation, because of seeing death coming in from the edges of abstraction where those with the luxury of time have cast it. I imagine what it would be like if friends had a demonstration each time a lover or a friend *or a stranger* died of AIDS. I imagine what it would be like if, each time a lover, friend *or stranger* died of this disease, their friends, lovers or neighbors would take the dead body and drive with it in a car a hundred miles an hour to washington d.c. and blast through the gates of the white house and come to a screeching halt before the entrance and dump their lifeless form on the front steps. It would be comforting to see those friends, neighbors, lovers *and strangers,* mark time and place and history in such a public way. (*CK*, 122; emphases added)

Here, to emphasize what is perhaps obvious, there is a strict inversion, a strict perversion, of the work of mourning. First, the very distinction between public and private, central to so much political theory, has been upset. What had been an essentially domestic ritual, part of a larger ritual system of domestication ensuring the "apolitical" privacy of domesticity, becomes a public, political act. The funeral, as a private ritual basically reserved for family, friends, and acquaintances of the dead, for the domus, that is to say, works as a kind of binding to guarantee the integrity and coherence, the shared affectivity and sentiment, of a community, a binding that thereby constitutes the *sensus communis* of the "community": the funeral would be the guarantee of identity.

But in Wojnarowicz, and this is my second point, the figure of the stranger is central. To introduce the stranger, either as "subject" or "object," to the funeral constitutes the eruption of the social in the field of a politics of the domestic community. As in the erotic, so too here, the stranger embodies that unbinding which is the social as the infinite proliferation of promiscuous, anonymous singularities: the stranger is not Everyman, but anyone. To mourn the stranger, which is necessarily always also to mourn *as* a stranger, is to engage the very existentiality or historicity of singularity. The proper name of the stranger, as in the recitation of names at displays of the AIDS quilt, or at observances of Kristalnacht, does not fix the stranger in an identity (and thus allows of no identification as sympathy or empathy), but is fundamentally an anonym. The anonym of the proper name is an attention to, as it articulates, the punctuality of whatever singularity. Like AIDS quilt panels that incorporate fetishes of the dead (or, more generally, emblems that a life was lived), the anonym is not a synecdoche that would express and represent the psychological integral unity of a subject. Rather, the anonym, the fetish, and the emblem are all metonymies standing for the impossibility of speaking the truth of beings in their whatever singularity; the "predicates," which would be the name, the fetish, the emblem, bespeak in fact the limit, the exhaustion of predication. At this limit, where the impossibility of saying is all that can be said, the social in its essential nonreserve appears in the "brief peek" of the heterogeneity of the "probable existence of literally millions of tribes." The figure of the stranger figures the punctuality of the social in its historicity.

And it does so with greatest attention to the force of outside, to existentiality, when the stranger is that intimate stranger which is both any and every dead body. The corpse, we have seen in reading Takenishi and Ōta, is at once that impossible figure or image which is the condition of possibility for the work of mourning, for historicization and ideality altogether; *and* the very nontranscendence of materiality in its utter abjection that is the surplus or excess of intersubjectivity and Imaginary identity. What would accumulate on the steps of the White House, at the rate of five bodies per hour at the time I am writing, would not only be the most material testimony to government inattention and callousness, but witness to the essential incapacity of the State to acknowledge the noncontainment or unbinding that is erotic sociality; no less is this the case at every display of the AIDS quilt or the recitation of names on Kristalnacht. This is testimony, a marking of "time and place and history," to that which every historicization necessarily occludes, the punctuation that gives the lie to every narrativization. Testimony to the limit of every positivist historiography, this is nevertheless, indeed thereby, testimony to the fact that there is history, to history in its historicity.

Now it was on the basis of Wojnarowicz's example, Jack Ben-Levi writes, that ACT UP adopted the practice of the political funeral in 1992; the major difference was that ACT UP deposited the cremated remains of the dead, rather than corpses, on the White House lawn: *feu la cendre*, indeed. As with the political funeral, so, too, many of Wojnarowicz's imagined actions are closely linked (whatever served as example or model for whomever) to various actions undertaken by groups such as ACT UP, the Lesbian Avengers, OutRage, Queer Nation, and so forth. In each action, undertaken to speak to a presumptively discrete incident or policy, or to make visible a particularly brutal practice or statement on the part of the government (for example), what appears in and as such singular interventions or disruptions is the heterogeneity of the social. Such actions will inevitably seem, from the perspective of the regulative protocols of the preinvented world, to be both unconscionably perverse (rather than merely criminal) and thereby violently terrorist, precisely because such actions are oriented toward a futurity substantially different than the present, a futurity to which consciousness is necessarily inadequate. This thought of such a futurity is the thought of a truly revolutionary, necessarily violent, and indeed cruel, change.

The Cruelty of the Ethical

"I have always been attracted to dangerous men, men whose gestures intimated the possibilities of violence, and I have always seduced them into states of gentle grace with my hands and lips" (*CK*, 271). It is a matter, then, of a violence, or rather the image or threat of violence, that will resonate simultaneously in the erotic, social, and political registers, none of which will occupy the prior ground of the ontological. But let us first consider violence, its image and threat, as it figures in the erotic. Consider the episode recorded in the section entitled "Doing Time in a Disposable Body" in *Memories That Smell Like Gasoline* (27–31). The narrator is picked up in a diner by an "intense and oddly sexy" deaf mute, "with a muscular body covered in scrapes and a few bruises," who "looked like he just walked out of some waterfront in an old queer french novel." *Querelle* perhaps? In any event, the reference is already to an Imaginary.

There was an air of desperation and possible violence around him like a rank perfume. And that was what suddenly became sexy to me. I tried to understand this sensation, why the remote edge of violence attracts me to a guy. I associate with certain gestures or body language or scars or other physical characteristics an entire flood of memories and fictions and mythologies. It's something in the blue-ink tattoos or coal-scratched rubbings made in prison cells or in delinquent basement parties. Maybe it's the sense that he could easily and dispassionately murder someone or rob a liquor store or a small roadside gas station or bang some salesman in the head at a highway rest stop and steal his automobile; it's something about the sense of violence carried as a distancing tool to break down the organized world. It's the weird freedom in his failure to recognize the manufactured code of rules. The violence that floats like static electricity that completely annihilates the possibility of future or security; I'm attracted to living like that, moment to moment, with very little piling up of information, breaking the windows of cause and response. Beyond all this it's also what happens when violence hangs above the road to the sexual act, that gets subverted within the series of small kissing motions at the base of my dick or across the underside of my balls. The sweetness of the sad lips of the criminal face lowering itself around my dick and the quiet sucking motion that I guide him into. It is not just that violence fades into sweetness; it's looking at the flesh of the body and recognizing that it is a restraint that keeps the blood inside the form; where the blood of the body creates a pressure so that it would spray out in every direction if it were not for the skin holding

it back; it's sensing the history of that body and the temporariness of
it all. I understand that his body and mind have no understanding of
the proscriptions [*sic*] of this society's values; that time is lost to him
except for progressions of gestures that attempt to satiate hungers of
various sorts. When I engage with a guy like this I am laying open a
trust, illusory or otherwise, that can strip open all the body's desires,
and for a brief moment of living we let ourselves get lost. (*MSG*,
27–30)

The deaf mute then attempts to pick the narrator's pockets during
sex and begins to get rough; the narrator responds with violence
and makes his escape into a departing subway train: what is sexy
here is the image of the possibility of violence. The realization of
that possibility, however, interrupts the sexual encounter and disrupts the erotic Imaginary. Thus, it is not violence "itself" that is
erotic, but the edge or *possibility* of transgressing a boundary; the
outlaw, perhaps obviously, is the embodiment of what the preinvented world must at all costs occlude, because its very existence
depends upon occlusion of that violence which is its very condition of possibility. The figure of the outlaw, stranger to any liberal
adjudication of private interests, figures the very instability or chaos
that any transgression of boundaries would disclose. A romantic,
perhaps masculinist figure, the outlaw. Most assuredly. But what
bears emphasis here is that the outlaw, a stranger whose possibilities we can imagine only in silhouette, as it were, and who is thus
the very figure of a truly radical contingency, who could in fact be
the other that is our death, is he who figures violence as the revelation of the absolute separation of the utter destitution of being, the
criminal impossibility of a being-in-common. This revelation is
aletheic: violence is truth, the truth of being (*CK*, 172–74). Violence is the aletheic revelation of the ontologically inhospitable
world, intolerable because inescapable. Violence discloses the essential cruelty of being, and it is the *threat*, or image, or possibility,
rather than the realization of that truth that is sexy. And this threat is
imagined or figured in a metonymic congeries of disparate signifiers: gestures, scars, movements, tattoos, charcoal rubbings, scrapes
and bruises, for example; in the very fragmentation of signification.

The threat or possibility of violence, which "floats like static electricity," the erotic charge, is that which *itself* "completely annihilates the possibility of future or security" and reduces the narrator to living "moment to moment" in the punctuality of infinite singularities. This reduction constitutes an existential *epochē*, the possibility that the "future" is the absence of future that is futurity. Which implies the impossibility of narrativity, most particularly (and this is the sexual/erotic charge) of a narrative of teleological orgasm. In this temporal syncope, this suspension of the narrative, sex becomes necessarily perverse, no longer organized and determined by a future. The encounter with the deaf mute is, in fact, interrupted: orgasm is unachieved. The body of the outlaw is indeed the incarnation of a radical historicity, because the temporality of the outlaw's "body" is that of an infinite fragmentation of gestures, which in their seeming immediacy never coalesce into the intentionality of a willing subject oriented toward a future project. Here, perhaps, the stranger is nothing other than the sheer weight of his animality; but it is nevertheless the case that it is with "a guy like this" that an absolute vulnerability, a trust, a loving—albeit "illusory"—becomes possible; there, in the threat of a violence to which one makes oneself vulnerable, it is possible to lose oneself.

This possibility or edge of violence, which carries such an erotic charge, resonates at once in both the erotic and political registers, for this eroticization of the possibility or edge of violence of which the outlaw is the figure, is always articulated in relation to the Law (the Law here signifying simultaneously the logos, as the condition of possibility for any intelligibility whatsoever, and the discursive regulation of bodies and practices—the "State"). It is in a negative relation to the Law, and in the very negativity of that relation, that the narrator situates himself: "Since my existence is essentially outlawed before I even come into knowledge of what my desires are or what my sensibility is, then I can only step back from the arms of government and organized religion and use similar techniques to walk from *here* to *there*" (*CK*, 59). Thus, "[r]ealizing that I have nothing left to lose in my actions I let my hands become weapons, my teeth become weapons, every bone and muscle and

fiber and ounce of blood become weapons, and I feel prepared for
the rest of my life" (*CK*, 81). It is the very negativity of the relation
to the Law that has always already outlawed him that the narrator
eroticizes: "The seductiveness of everything the State finds repellant or threatening to its structure always draws me back to examine
it, at least until I see its shape" (*CK*, 217). Ben-Levi is undoubtedly
right to argue that all this is to eroticize the agency of repression itself. Yet it is also necessary to recognize, as Ben-Levi in fact does,
that much more than the question of utopian liberation is at stake
here.

From the perspective of we Wojnarowiczes, who have always
already been *identified*, by the Law and in law, as being "in our being" outlaws (and it is still open season on queers in many places), it
is the legality of the Law, including the very rationality of the logos,
that is at stake. From this perspective, the very legality of the Law is
arbitrary: "We're told not to cross certain lines, and yet those lines
are crossed every day by those in power" (*CK*, 234–35). Of course,
such a remark can be read to be merely a comment on the willful
failure of those in power to respect the rule of Law; but that does
not address the question of what makes such abuse *possible*. In other
words, transgression or criminality is possible if—and only if—we
admit the arbitrariness of the Law itself. No transgression or criminality is possible with respect to what is called the law of gravity;
but the Law as State or as logos is ultimately unjustifiable in the
sense of being arbitrary, and therefore anarchic in its ground. Furthermore, the Law (for example, the State) is the occlusion of the
instituting violence of which law is the institution; the Law is—in
itself and as such—illegal, a fact it must conceal at all costs. It is the
figure of the outlaw in Wojnarowicz that reveals the essential violence of the Law, because it is the "criminal" each of us ultimately
is (in our heterogeneous singularities) that provokes the Law's every
exercise of violence.

From this perspective, to imagine the possibility of violence is
to imagine the possibility of difference, the possibility *for* difference.
Which does not amount to a utopianism, because what is imagined
here is not this or that particular alternative, but the fact of differ-

ence itself, which makes any alternative imaginable. What is being imagined is the possibility that there is history, that there is that to which everything imaginable is utterly and essentially inadequate, a radically incommensurable difference. Unless there is that which opens upon the essential instability, insecurity, and danger of a futurity that can never be the telos of a project, unless one encounters the outlaw as that risk, surprise, or indeed ruin that is the existential, then one can only confirm the Law in its presumptive connaturality. Without the possibility that anything goes, then nothing goes—let alone comes. And here is the possibility for concerted social action oriented toward a futurity immanent, and imminent, in any future: "Rage may be one of the few things that binds or connects me to you, to our preinvented world" (*CK*, 117). This, then, would be to enact a sociality established in the difference of the separation of radical singularities; it would therefore open upon the possibility of politicality as such, a possibility entirely foreclosed in Wojnarowicz's preinvented world. In this sense, political historiography, however informal, traces the prehistory of a politicality yet to be realized.

The relation of the outlaw, always already confirmed in the essential criminality of what is taken to be his identity, to the Law, is one of sovereignty. This sovereignty is not to be construed as the autonomy of the outlaw who is a "law unto himself," for the sovereignty of the figure of the outlaw in its negativity calls into question the possibility for any nomos whatever. Neither, therefore, can this sovereignty, which is a sovereign *loss* or abandonment of "self," be reduced to any egoism; and this is where Wojnarowicz's sovereignty breaks with every romanticism. The sovereign figure of the outlaw is neither hero nor anti-hero; there is no triumph of the will, no courage or even audacity, which would be the attribute of a being, here, precisely because the erotic, and the threat of violence, which is an opening upon the erotic, does not refer to any experiential unity of a psychological subject; the possibility of violence is not a *frisson* befalling the integrity of an autoaffectivity. Rather, sovereignty must be taken here to be the nonpositive affirmation (nonpositive because it is neither predicate, attribute, nor quality) of the limit-experience, where power or force is the very

absence of ground of the political; it is the nonpositive affirmation
of the absolute separation of whatever singularities, of being in its
essential ruin or destitution, in its unjustifiability, of the violence
that being *is* in its be-ing. This is the nonpositive affirmation of
Ōta's Gin-chan, of the narrator of John Rechy's *City of Night*, of
Joey in Samuel R. Delany's *Tale of Plagues and Carnivals*, of "Jean
Genet," of Wojnarowicz's Dakota (*CK*, 165–276).[70] Sovereignty is
at once oriented toward futurity and the threat of violence that is
the stranger, the outlaw; sovereignty, therefore, is essentially vulnerability, and as such opens upon the question of the ethical.

The ethical here has nothing to do with aspirations to be a
good person (either as achievement or as failure, the ontological
stain that is the "sinner"); nor is the ethical here even a matter of
"doing the right thing." In both cases, we would, of course, have to
assume at least the ideal possibility of a transcendental perspective
from which judgments might be made. Indeed, the ethical may well
be neither predicate, attribute, nor quality of being or acts. It might
well be impossible to say what the ethical *is*, or in what ethicality
might reside. One cannot say what the ethical is, beyond a question it is almost impossible, but nonetheless necessary, to pose. Perhaps, in fact, the ethical may well be acknowledgment of the essential impossibility of saying what the ethical might be. The ethical
would therefore be originarily aporetic, a question impossible to
pose but that nevertheless demands a response: the most practical
of exigencies. The ethical would therefore reside in the demand to
pose the question of the ethical. Whatever. But, and this is the
point, the ethical dimension would be forever occluded and foreclosed were it not for the thought of the absolute nontranscendence
of what I have called sovereignty, the figure that is the nonpositive
affirmation of historicity, sociality, politicality. The aporia of the
ethical can only appear in the disjunction between the Law and that
which it excludes. We can only think that there is the aporia of the
ethical if we can figure or imagine the difference between, for example, "the State and the unbinding which it prohibits" (Agamben), between the preinvented world (in and as its inscription) and
that which it occludes.

The Erotic Praxis of Poiesis

So it is a question in Wojnarowicz of the possibility, of the edge, of the figure, of the image of that disjunction; it might well be argued that this writing is the production of that disjunction, that which is both produced by that disjunction and conversely produces it, both witness to that disjunction (testimony) and a practice (as enactment) of that disjunction, a disjunction we might therefore call history. It is in any case in the first instance a matter of possibilities, of the edge, of the figure, of the image of the violence of that disjunction; neither Jacobin Imaginary nor Sorelian myth, this image is the figure of the immanence of the violence of be-ing, but it is indeed, as Ben-Levi stresses, a "fantasized violence."[71] Wojnarowicz himself repeatedly emphasized the Imaginary, figural aspect of this violence throughout *Close to the Knives*, as well as in an interview with Adam Kuby.[72] Nevertheless, the figure or image of violence is most disturbing, not when it purports to be merely the record of the violence-in-general of the "world," but when it is thought to express a "repellant *intent*"; thus, a drawing of violence is more disturbing to many people than a photograph of violence (*CK*, 184). In response to objections to representations of promiscuous, "unsafe" sex, Wojnarowicz wrote:

> I'm beginning to believe that one of the last frontiers left for radical gesture is the imagination. At least in my ungoverned imagination I can fuck somebody without a rubber, or I can, in the privacy of my own skull, douse Helms with a bucket of gasoline and set his putrid ass on fire or throw congressman William Dannemeyer off the empire state building. These fantasies give me distance from my outrage for a few seconds. They give me momentary comfort. Sexuality defined in images gives me comfort in a hostile world. They give me strength.
> (*CK*, 120)

Something more than a safety-valve, functionalist, conception of fantasy is at work here, and that something more is the vision of the violence, the destitution, the ultimate entropy or indifference of being, which is the unacknowledged ground of the preinvented Other World. An unimagined or unfigured violence, as our histories demonstrate very well, of itself produces no disjunction; it is only insofar as it can be thought, albeit as the unthinkable, or imagined, albeit as the unimaginable, or figured, albeit as the unfigurable, that violence, or radical historicity, can *figure* difference. In short, whatever the specific image in this fantasized violence, the image is ultimately the image of the corpse, of the fact that there is history, the image of the "il y a" or "Es gibt" of historicity. Without this figure of the body of this death—in other words, "historical consciousness"—any praxis oriented toward a future substantially different from the present would be unimaginable. Something other than *Einbildungskraft* (because it is the imagining of the possibility of Einbildungskraft), this constitutes an erotic poiesis, an erotics of thought.

> I discovered that making things meant leaving evidence of life behind when I moved on. Making things was like leaving historical records of my existence behind when I left the room, or building, or neighborhood, the state and possibly the earth . . . as in mortality, as in death. When I was a kid I discovered that making an object, whether it was a drawing or a story, meant making something that spoke even if I was silent. As an adult, I realize if I make something and leave it in public for any period of time, I can create an environment where that object or writing acts as a magnet and draws others with a similar frame of reference out of silence or invisibility. (*CK*, 156)

What is at stake here is, not the creation of artifacts or of an oeuvre, a personal accomplishment, but rather a gesture or movement, of which that which is made is no more, but no less, than the trace of its making. It is for this reason, perhaps, that Wojnarowicz could recall in an interview with Barry Blinderman:

> I remember that I would buy grass seed and walk around inside the warehouse, down near Canal Street and throw this grass seed all over. All the disintegrated plaster that had fallen out of the ceiling and all the airborne particles of earth and stuff would actually let this grass grow in the confines of the building, so it would be like an actual meadow inside several rooms that were just so beautiful. I got the idea for that because one day I saw mushrooms growing in some of the rooms and I thought, well if mushrooms grow, then maybe grass

seed will, too. Those are some of the gestures that I loved the most and got the least attention because they were the most anonymous—you couldn't sign a blade of grass that says Wojnarowicz.[73]

What is made then, is the trace of a poiesis, figuration, a "historical record" of the fact of poiesis, the fact *that there is* poiesis; what is made testifies to its referent, certainly, but more important to the fact that it was made, *to the praxis of its poiesis*, that is to say. And it is this witness ("to existence," as Wojnarowicz writes) that draws others, readers, for example, "out of silence or invisibility." This makes of Wojnarowicz's writing a call, a summons, a demand for attention to the disjunction between the preinvented Other World, which subsists in the nondisclosure of its ground, and the apocalyptic historicity that is an ultimate absence of ground.

In the "Postscript" to "The Suicide of a Guy Who Once Built an Elaborate Shrine over a Mousehole," the narrator goes to the bullfights, "hoping the sight of blood would shake me up and wake me up to all that which had no words" (*CK*, 257–58): "Behind us, far over the walls of the arena, the vague notes of the band begin again and float like thin banners across the hot sky. Meat. Blood. Memory. War. We rise to greet the State, to confront the State. Smell the flowers while you can" (*CK*, 276).

Y su sangre ya viene cantando. . . .

CHAPTER 6

Second Excursus on the Divine Right
of the Historian

The engraving stylus of history depicts him only when he makes
himself seen, but then it is not he.

—Comte Donatien-Alphonse-François de Sade,
Les Crimes de l'amour

Ecce Homo will have given us this to think about: History or historical science, which puts to death or treats the dead, which deals
or negotiates with the dead, is the science of the father. It occupies the place of the dead and the place of the father.

—Jacques Derrida, *The Ear of the Other*

This second excursus on the divine right of the historian is
concerned, as in a sense this entire investigation has been, with the
extraordinary onto-epistemological privilege accorded the historian
situated at the conjunction of a rhetorical invocation of "history itself" with an unreflective or nothing-but-reflective anthropocentrism. The coincidence of a "historical consciousness" that refuses to
think the thought of its own limits with an anthropocentric historicism, a modern subjectivity that admits of no alterity and
thereby purports to achieve identity, is a conjunction that has been
under attack for rather a long time now from a number of different
perspectives. What I want to pursue here is the pertinence of
Tanizaki Jun'ichirō's *Busshū kō hiwa* (*The Secret History of the Lord of
Musashi*) to a critique of any conflation of a concept of history as

the continuity of unities (which are construed to find their very unity in the seminal inspiration of a virile originality) with a concept of identity construed as the intersubjective recognition of essential similitude. In other words, I am concerned with whether the enabling protocols of every appeal to the tumescent plenitude of the modern subject of history are in fact protocols that are themselves phallogocentric, irrespective of the objects studied or the explicitly expressed politics of any given representation of those objects. Also at issue, therefore, will be the question of whether it is possible to situate any "historical" discourse entirely "outside" of phallogocentric discourse in the name of, or for the sake of, any critical politics.

I argue that the pertinence of Tanizaki's *Secret History* is a question of a parody that is no mere irony, a question of staging, a question of performativity. The *Secret History* first appeared serially in 1931–32 in the magazine *Shinseinen* (New Youth); it was revised, provided with what is for us a very important preface, and published in book form in 1935.[74] The text of the *Secret History* closes with the observation that in committing to writing the disclosures that comprise his text, the author intended that subsequent perusals of official histories such as the *Tsukuma gunki* (Military Records of the Tsukuma), the text that presents the protagonists of the *Secret History* in the carapaces of their public subject positions, would lead to the discovery of unexpected perspectives. In calling for reading as what Paul Ricoeur once termed with reference to Freud a "hermeneutics of suspicion," whoever or whatever we are taking the "author" to be marks the text of the *Secret History* as first and foremost a parody of the *monumental* historiography—the *monumenta Nipponica*—of the official chronicles.

Here, a brief reference to Foucault's reading of Nietzsche's untimely meditation on monumental history seems pertinent.[75] Recall, briefly, Nietzsche's characterization of monumental history, a history made by the "man of deeds and power" whose persona is so large and forceful that it can only be described in terms of excess: the very portrait of the heroic subject. To those who view the monumental history made by such a man, his deeds and power project an image in the mirror of history that is "worthy of imitation," a heroism that is always "possible a second time." The great danger, as Marx had already seen, is that subjective identity achieved in the historical Imaginary of monumental historiography can end in unconsciously parodic farce. Or, as Nietzsche wrote, "monumental history deceives by analogies" and "seductive similarities," engendering a facile specular identification, one sense in which for Nietzsche the past can suffocate the present.[76] But monumental history not only engenders parody, Foucault stresses, but can itself be parodic. As parody, it "opposes the themes of recognition or reminiscence,"[77] and can itself become the carnivalesque play of masquerade. And in Foucault, of course, the masquerade of a parodic monumental history is one of the major dimensions of genealogy as a disseminatory practice of the palimpsest, and is therefore linked to the question of the origin, to the historicist construction of identity, and to the consequent authority of knowledge. The origin, which always "lies at a place of inevitable loss, the point where the truth of things corresponds to a truthful discourse,"[78] is the always already occluded site where the saying and the said would putatively be identical, where parody would therefore be impossible. It is only in a genealogy that forgoes the search for origins that parody is possible. Which renders illusory and fantasmatic man's search for the continuity and similitude that would confirm his identity and subjectivity in history. Concomitantly, historical knowing can no longer in any sense be an authorization of the exercise of power. Now, whatever the status of Foucault's essay as a prescription for historiography, it links the parody of the monumental to questions of the establishment of anthropocentric identity and to the authorization of the exercise of power under the aegis of history. Indeed, it is that essentially parodic genealogy, History in drag, that threatens both the virile originality of a subjectivity that finds its identity in the mirror of history and a "destructive aggressivity" exercised in the name of knowledge.

Staging the Seen, the Unseen, and the Obscene

I shall delay for a while a discussion of the essentially parodic poiesis by which Tanizaki stages the text of the *Secret History*; at the outset, however, it is important to note that it is in part presented to us as a series of tableaux—a chronicle rather than a narrative history—set in the sixteenth century, a period historiography has traditionally termed the "era of warring states" (*sengoku jidai*). Often enough, historians have referred to the sixteenth century as an age of "chaos" or of disorder, an outlaw period, constituted as the outside of properly historical reason largely because the putative unities according to which historiography constructs its proper rationality—the "nation-state" in particular—are missing or lacking. In any case, the text presents a series of tableaux, in each of which the structure of a secret masochistic desire and the achievement of a visible public persona or subject-position through a dialectic of intersubjective recognition are strictly isomorphic. It is this isomorphism that I want briefly to investigate in each of four tableaux.

The "Lord of Musashi," whom I hesitate to call hero, anti-hero, protagonist, or even actant for reasons I hope will become clear, is twelve years old at the opening of the first scene and is known by his childhood name, Hōshimaru. He has been raised as a hostage in the castle of a lord who once bested Hōshimaru's father in battle and to whom Hōshimaru's father has therefore sworn fealty and acknowledged subservience. As the hostage of a rivalry between territorial lords, Hōshimaru is therefore himself the visible sign or token of a provisional and tentative resolution of a life-and-death struggle among masters; he is himself the token of the recognition of an intersubjective relation between lord and bondsman. I should emphasize, however, that from any Hegelian perspective, this relation, because it is never overcome in the Kojèvian poiesis of the bondsman's labor,[79] remains a relation of domination *within* a society of masters, and it can therefore never become "historical"; Hōshimaru is *also* therefore a token of exchange that signifies the *impossibility* of any final resolution of rivalry within a society of masters.

The year is 1549 and Ojika Castle, where Hōshimaru is being

raised as hostage, is under siege. Because he is only twelve years old (and *not* because he is a hostage), Hōshimaru is allowed neither to participate in nor to witness the scene of battle. He is chagrined and humiliated because he is granted no participatory public persona or subject-position; indeed, he is humiliated because he has never once been spattered with blood or even seen the fragmented, mutilated body of a warrior. An older woman of the samurai class therefore undertakes to reveal the scene of his destiny within the signifying order (that is to say, within the *domus*) to him, a scene wherein he will achieve the subject-positionality of the samurai's public persona; swearing Hōshimaru to secrecy, she undertakes to reveal to him his identity and fate *as* a samurai, the telos of his public ambition, the presumptive meaning of his being. For what she reveals to him is the scene where severed heads taken in battle are washed and dressed in order to be presented to the Gaze of the lord and master as visible evidence of the destructive and therefore virile aggressivity of his retainers. Hōshimaru is confident that he is prepared for all this.

What takes him completely by surprise, however, is that this revelation of the presumptive meaning of his public being is at the same time the advent of his erotic desire, the unveiling of the scene of his fantasies. The two are not the same, but they intersect at every point and are strictly symmetrical. The destructive aggressivity, the sadism, of his public persona is reflected in the scene of erotic desire, which is in all respects that of classical masochism. It is precisely the protocols of the signifying order of his public persona that determine the limits or frame of Imaginary possibility for him: the structure of his desire is an effect of his position within the signifying order. Four points seem to be particularly pertinent here:

1. It is a matter of specular capture. What as an object of fascination focuses his gaze is precisely the objectness of the severed heads; these heads are *nothing but* objects to be subjected to the manipulation of the women who are washing and dressing them. And the more abject these objects are, the better: the manipulation at the hands of a beautiful woman of old, ugly, or mutilated heads arouses his desire in a much more disturbing manner than the ma-

nipulation of the heads of handsome young samurai. But he is also the more aroused the more successfully he can identify himself as *being* the abject object. To be at the side of the women in itself excites him not at all; he must perceive himself to have been killed and decapitated. He must see his severed head being seen and manipulated by the women. He can desire only insofar as he "is" the abject object of the Gaze. Indeed, he must say to himself "Jibun de aru"—"that is me" (or, perhaps better, "It is myself" or "It is the self"). But of course, Hōshimaru realizes that aspiration to such an identification is a contradiction (*mujun*), for if he actually *were* that utterly abject object, a corpse, he would have no consciousness, thus forfeiting the pleasure of seeing himself being seen in the scene. And so he realizes that it is the staging of a scene, the *re*presentation in fantasy that is itself the pleasure, for clearly it is a representation that can represent no original located in the Real. Central to his masochism, therefore, is not only the specular identification of himself in the abjection of being nothing-but-object but also the mastery of being able to stage, manipulate, and witness the scene of his own abjection.

2. The scene is most erotic for Hōshimaru as the figural or Imaginary *representation of* castration; what is in question here is not castration as that which befalls the phallus as it supposedly "is" either penis or clitoris, but the phallus as the simulacrum of a tumescent virility. Thus, the mutilated heads are most fascinating when the nose is missing. The missing nose of a corpse is in itself a sign of the victor's aggressivity, for the nose is a synecdoche for the head, just as the head is a synecdoche for the body. And one does not need to have read the Freud/Fliess correspondence to recognize the nose to be phallic: noseless heads are called "woman-heads" in the *Secret History* (*onna kubi*). Further on, indeed, there is some question of whether a nose preserved in red ink is in fact a nose or another, equally pulpy protuberance: the narrator's discretion draws a veil over the fact of the matter, thus reinforcing the phallic status of the "nose."

3. Hōshimaru's fantasies and fascinations are always subject to a certain osculation. They either entirely usurp the scene of what is

here taken to be actuality, or they are *occluded by* that actuality. Even though actuality and fantasy present the "same" images, the actual and fantastic statuses of those images are mutually exclusive; once fantasy is recognized to be actual, desire is lost. The actual, however immediate and actual it may in fact *be*, must be transfigured into fantasy in order to be the scene of desire. Revelation of actuality (or the unveiling of the phallus) marks the end of erotic satisfaction. Indeed: what could possibly ever be erotic about a cigar that is only a cigar?

4. Hōshimaru's desire commits him to an obsessive compulsion to repeat, to stage in an endless repetition the specularity of the spectacle of his masochistic desire. I shall come back to this point; suffice it to notice for now that Hōshimaru, both in his public ambition and in his secret desire, is condemned to a repetition of the Same (in the banal sense and in the sense of banality), and concomitantly that the scene of Hōshimaru's desire is one that admits of no alterity—because even if he is the object for another, he himself stages the scene of fantasy.

According to the narrator, so obsessed is Hōshimaru with restaging the scene of his desire that he surreptitiously returns every night to watch heads being washed and dressed, always by the same women and always in the same way. Presently, inevitably, as the ferocity of battle abates, he is faced with an absence of severed heads, and in particular with "woman heads." He undertakes to remedy the situation by sneaking into the enemy camp and decapitating and mutilating a samurai; the head will then be brought to the women to dress and he will be able to gaze once again upon his fantasy. But things go too well. He kills the enemy commander, takes his nose, kills two of his pages and sneaks back in to Ojika Castle, a deed that will remain forever an enigma to all the combatants, and its perpetrator unacknowledged in the official histories. Leaderless and insulted, the enemy lift the siege and depart; thus, although Hōshimaru has learned the erotic pleasure of destructive aggressivity and has in fact performed the first of many feats that will delineate his heroic public persona, from the perspective of his immediate aim, the adventure has been disastrous. What is important here, I think, is the intersection of what will be his public life with his secret desires. The narrator goes so far in his hermeneutics of suspicion as to suggest that public ambition and subject-positionality are always determined by personal psychological motives. But it is equally important to observe that nowhere in the text are we offered an *etiology* of Hōshimaru's masochism; neither his ambition nor his desire is thus assigned an *origin* that would be thought to explain either or both. In the sense that public ambition and a secret desire intersect in their symmetrical structures, but are irreducible to each other or to a singular *origin*, then, their relation is one of an ultimately undecidable oscillation. In any case, the narrator informs us that two years later, Hōshimaru comes of age, takes his adult name, Terukatsu, and is entirely absorbed in his public ambitions for some years.

The third scene I want to mention constitutes the longest, most complex narrative section of the *Secret History* and deserves an extended analysis in itself. But to cut, as it were, a long story short, it details Terukatsu's political and erotic involvement with one "Lady Kikyō," daughter of the enemy commander slain and relieved of his nose by Hōshimaru, who is haunted by the vengeful ghost of her father. Seeking revenge for her dead and mutilated father, she marries Norishige, heir of the lord to whom Terukatsu owes fealty, and whom she holds responsible for her father's humiliation. Kikyō and Terukatsu enter into a literally labyrinthine political and erotic conspiracy to deprive Norishige of his nose; she in order to exact political revenge, Terukatsu in order to see a live but noseless Norishige *in camera* with Kikyō, a restaging of the scene of desire. Numerous abortive attempts are made on Norishige's nose. Successively, his lip is cut (not only disfiguring his face but impeding his speech), he loses an ear (thus depriving his face of specular symmetry), and finally the nose is taken in a virtually surgical maneuver. This has a number of consequences beyond satisfying the more or less immediate respective goals of Kikyō and Terukatsu:

1. Norishige's castration—and it *is* castration in every sense except the explicitly genital—is the result of a specifically political treachery carried out by a wife to whom he was married as a political alliance and with the sanction of the shogun, in complicity with

a retainer whose first obligation was presumptively loyalty to his lord. Thus, the fact that henceforth Norishige refuses to be seen by all but his most senior retainers and confines himself to the women's quarters is more than a personal shyness or embarrassment over what is quite literally a "loss of face." It marks his loss of political authority and presence, the precipitous decline of his political power. No longer does Norishige swagger in the company of his retainers; he necessarily retreats from his dominant and dominating position in the virile rivalry of the phratry. This loss of the political presence of Norishige's persona becomes absolute with the loss of his domain itself and the murder of his son and heir; the genealogical series that always repeats the virile originality of the generation of the seminal inspiration is cut off and, indeed, annihilated.

2. Norishige's consecutive mutilations bring about the end of his celebrations of the presence of the enunciative voice in song and poetry recitation. Once proud of his voice in signing and lyric poetry, Norishige's voice is increasingly "crippled," to the point where his words become unintelligible. The authentic voice of the ancient Japanese poets is cut off in castration. Norishige therefore turns to the *writing* of poetry; it is castration that opens for him onto the absence of presence that *is* the writing that is in *all* language. This castration, this spacing or distance, which is the absence of presence, opens for Norishige onto difference and historicity, and onto difference *as* historicity. I shall return to this.

3. More immediately, Norishige's castration introduces the radical nonimmediacy, the essential displacement and supplementarity, of intertextuality. Specifically, for the first and only time in the *Secret History*, there is reference to a text that exists "outside" of the *Secret History* itself. Kikyō puns at a poetry-writing session on a poem in the *Genji monogatari* entitled "The Village of Falling Blossoms." (The pun is that in Japanese *hana* is a homophone signifying both blossom and nose.) Thus, castration opens not only upon writing, intertextuality, and historicity, but also cuts the signifier loose from the signified, giving the lie to the presumptive transcendentality of the signified. Small wonder, then, that Terukatsu, trapped in the endless repetition of the fantasy of the presence of his own absence and

therefore captive of the illusion of phallic presence itself, is hard put to read the "message" encoded in Kikyō's reference and misses the intertextuality of the reference entirely. I shall come back to the further complications of this question of intertextuality.

4. Because castration opens upon historicity, it also and thereby opens on to an impossibility for historical representation. Again, I want to come back to this point later; here, I merely want to note that Norishige's castration—which is not a genital one—completely alters the relation between Kikyō and her husband. For she finds that with the removal of Norishige's nose (and consequently the assumption of historicity as absence of presence), she has discharged her political responsibility to her father's ghost, the presence of his absence; that she is thereby freed from the Law of the Father; and that therefore, in short, she loves her husband. And this love, which emerges "outside the limits of the law, where alone it may live" as Lacan says, resists historical representation and knowing absolutely. But if castration means for Norishige and Kikyō an entirely different relation (and here the term "love" can only signify that difference), Terukatsu endlessly seeks to restage the scene of his subjectivity and desire.

The fourth scene I want to discuss is set in 1558, when Terukatsu, at twenty-one years of age, marries Shōsetsuin, who is fourteen. At first, for Terukatsu, this marriage is the most perfunctory of his obligations and at the furthest remove from his desire. The lack of attention from her husband upsets Shōsetsuin not at all. But Terukatsu undertakes a seduction, an introduction of Shōsetsuin to the scene of his desire—an introduction that in many respects mimics his own introduction to the scene nine years before. The central figure in this seduction is Terukatsu's servant Dōami. Dōami delights Shōsetsuin and her companions with the virtuosity of his mimicry, the enjoyment or fascination of which lies not in the realism of his representations, of course, for no one actually believes that Dōami is a firefly, for example, but rather in the very fact that his imitations *are* imitations. The real deception lies elsewhere. For Terukatsu pretends to take delight in Shōsetsuin's games and gradually leads her to take up a role in the staging of his own obsession. Dōami is thereupon ordered to present, to represent, the severed head of Terukatsu's fantasy, upon pain of performing the "role" in actuality. Thus, night after night, Dōami is required to remain absolutely motionless while at a few yards distance—a distance that only enhances the illusion—Terukatsu gazes upon Dōami's *apparently* severed head and takes his pleasure of his alternately giddy and terrified bride. Two points bear emphasis here. Dōami's function is to imitate the terror and anguish that he actually feels, for he must feign the fate that will be his in reality if he gives the lie to the representation of illusion. Second, Dōami's role is that of *le mort*, the Imaginary figure that, although the object of a masochistic subjective identification, is entirely at the mercy, or lack thereof, of him who stages the fantasy: Dōami is denied any alterity whatsoever. But Dōami is *le mort* in yet another sense of the term. For his function is also that of the dummy (or *le mort*) in bridge—he who lays all his cards on the table, cards that are dealt to him and will be played by his partner, but who himself does not play the game. If you have been reading Lacan, you will recognize here the figure of the psychoanalyst, he whose subject-position is always to be out of place, displaced, and therefore other *to* intersubjective identification. So it is no surprise that later it is Dōami to whom Terukatsu confesses the secret history of his desire; and it is in large part from *Dōami hanashi*—"talks of Dōami"—that the texts of *The Secret History of the Lord of Musashi* will be assembled.

In any case, Shōsetsuin becomes a nun at some unspecified later date; Dōami survives to write the *Dōami hanashi*; Terukatsu survives to the age of forty-two, endlessly reproducing the ob-scene of his desire with a promiscuous succession of women and "dummys"—all of whom, the narrator tells us, Terukatsu has put to death.

Three points, perhaps, bear recapitulation before continuing:

1. At all points, Terukatsu is entirely caught up in a "bad infinity." In terms of his public, ostensibly political subject-positionality, he is captive of a relation between lord and bondsman within which the mutual recognition of lord and bondsman never leads to a dialectical sublation (*Aufhebung*); the relation is one, therefore that obtains in a society of masters. Precisely because it is constituted in

a *non*dialectical relationality, Terukatsu's persona belongs to an order that resists all the teleologies—and not merely the Hegelian—of historical reason and comprehension. Concomitantly, neither is the sadomasochistic relation according to which Terukatsu stages the scene of his desire a dialectical relation. Least of all is it a dialogical relation. And this precisely because there is no intersubjectivity in the sadomasochistic fantasy, dedicated as it is to the nonrelationality of alterity. Furthermore, the relation between Terukatsu's persona and the construction of his sadomasochistic desire is itself *non*dialectical, thereby resisting the specific comprehensibility that historicization promises.

2. Norishige's castration, because it cuts him off from the virile originality and presence of the lyric voice, opens upon "writing" as the trace that *indicates* the absence of presence, upon the difference between the material signifier and the Imaginary signified (puns), upon an intertextuality as a relation among signifiers that is not constituted in a passage through the signifieds of the Imaginary, and finally upon "love"—a term that has no signification in the text other than its very resistance to any signified. In every respect, then, castration opens upon historicity as absence, difference, and spacing; in other words, upon what Lacan calls "language." Castration is the *impossibility* of presence, identity, and unity, the *impossibility* of what commonsense constitutes as the properly "historical."

3. As I have already mentioned, the text is set in the "premodern" sixteenth century, an "age" or "period" that, long characterized as one of "chaos" or "disorder," has constituted a kind of madness or insanity *without which* an anthropocentric historicism could never recognize itself, relieved and jubilant, to be the privileged locus of intelligibility, rationality, and identity. On all three points, then, we are dealing with the limits of a certain construction of what common sense takes to be a fundamentally unproblematic "historical consciousness."

These questions, which mark the aporiae of every straightforward notion of historical consciousness, are raised on at least two further levels of the construction of the *Secret History*. First, the *Secret History* purports to be just that, the revelation of the truth of a *se-*

cret history. ("Secret history" is the translator Anthony Chambers's rendering of *hiwa*—a secret or hidden, in any case veiled, speech or relation.) The narrator (whose fictive identity is never disclosed, but who is in no case Tanizaki Jun'ichirō "himself") undertakes to reveal that which official historiography has missed, or indeed, occluded. The narrator thus takes it upon himself (and there is good reason to assume the narrator is to be taken to be a man) to supplement and augment the historical record; he will fill in the gaps, performing one of the classical functions of historical research. But *also*, and *thereby*, the narrator, accomplished historian that he shows himself to be, stages a scene of intersubjective recognition between author and reader. For in claiming to reveal a heretofore secret history—a history that *is* secret, but also the secret *of* history—the narrator assumes an essential epistemological, and therefore ontological, similitude between himself and the reader. He tells the reader, as it were, that "together, you and I, we *are* the subject of historical knowing. We may disagree, you and I, over this or that, but we need not question the grounds of every possible agreement: we know, *mon semblable, mon frère*, what history is."

This revelation, a true relation of a heretofore secret history, is possible only because the narrator has privileged access to privately held documents, the objects of every proper historian's professional desire. And these documents or sources are memoirs by two former servants of Terukatsu's or of his near entourage. The first is "A Dream Seen of a Night," by a certain nun, Myōkaku. Of Myōkaku little is known, but the narrator finds textual evidence to suggest that she was at one time in the service of the lord of Musashi. (She might, in fact, although there is no evidence to support this conjecture, be Shōsetsuin.)[80] The narrator suggests that, as a presumptively celibate nun, Myōkaku wrote out of sexual frustration. The second document or source for the *Secret History* is the *Dōami hanashi*, "talks of Dōami," he of the psychoanalytic impasse, who wrote out of an inability to forget his past, and to whom Terukatsu confessed his secret history. So we recognize the narrator to be, very like ourselves, a good historian: not only has he grubbed around in the Kiryū family storehouse to bring new sources to the light of historical understanding, sources that themselves bring that which was absent into a presence to knowledge; he also treats these sources with a properly scholarly suspicion. The narrator unveils for us that which would bring us ever closer to the plenitude—the tumescence—of historical knowing. What we thought we had lost is restored to us. And it is precisely in this recuperation of the past that castration is revealed to have been but a bad dream, because this increase of knowledge is the guarantee of the presence and identity of the subjects of knowledge: nothing is lost. And it is just this that allows narrator and reader to recognize their essential similitude.

But this scene of intersubjective recognition, this reunion of men of knowledge in the phratry of an eminently sober scholarship, is staged itself by the text, and it is staged as parody. We generally conceive parody to be an "ironic imitation" of a wholly serious original; it is of course frequently the seriousness of the original that is parodied. And in order for the "irony"—the suspended subjectivity of the parodist, a kind of beautiful soul always in reserve—of the parody to be recognized, the imitation or mimesis of the parody must be marked *as such*. Otherwise, the satire, farce, or risibility of the parody falls flat. Parody only works if everyone gets the joke, if parodist and audience alike recognize, behind the play of parodic representation, a shared understanding, an intersubjectivity constituted in knowledge (of the "original," of a "style" or whatever). But there are further possibilities in parody, which pose a radical threat to the essential safety and reassurances of irony.

One of the reputed pleasures of parody when it is conceived as irony is the reassurance that it gives to those who "get the joke" that it is possible *not* to get the joke. In this sense, parody is always in some sense an attempted deception, a seduction. But parodic deception must always mark itself, in whatever way, to *be* in fact a deception; and insofar as it marks itself as "deception," it is *not* a deception, it tells the truth. As Foucault and Lacan among others have demonstrated, it says, "I am lying." Now the possibility of saying, "I am lying" indicates the possibility of a feigned deception: as long as the truth is outrageous enough, it will be taken to be a lie. And this marks the radical undecidability of any protest of veracity: it may be true, it may be a deception, it may be truth masquerading as deception, and so on, ad infinitum. But this is possible only because there is a difference between the subject of the *énonciation*—the saying of what is said—and the subject of the *énoncé*, the subject about which something is predicated. Which of course creates the possibility for every kind of ventriloquism, including irony and parody. (But notice that it is now impossible confidently to distinguish the ventriloquist from the dummy—or indeed, from that other dummy, *le mort*.) What in any case is at stake here is the "originary" displacement and supplementarity of the authorial voice, the originary displacement and supplementarity—but you see where I am headed—of the virile originality of lyrical ejaculation. In short: the parodic is the sign of castration.

Now, this entire congeries of questions is signaled at the very outset in the Preface to the *Secret History*. Well, not quite the outset, because the "Preface" is dated "early autumn" of Shōwa 10 (1935), after the rest of the text appeared in 1931–32. Of all the parodic marks that the text bears, it is this Preface in which the displacement and supplementarity of the authorial voice is unavoidable. While the rest of the *Secret History* is written in a straightforward modern Japanese, with a few archaic or pseudo-archaic locutions thrown in, the Preface is written in *kanbun*, the Japanese method of construing written Chinese. Until the latter part of the nineteenth century, *kanbun* was generally, if not always, the accepted mode in which the Japanese themselves wrote official documents, formal scholarly treatises, official histories, and the like. But with the exception of Sino-Japanese characters and a certain written vocabulary, the Chinese and Japanese languages have nothing in common. In particular, because the syntax of Japanese is very different from that of Chinese, it is necessary to rearrange the word order of every sentence according to a kind of road map, which often seems to indicate nothing but detours that must be negotiated before the syntagma can be enunciated. Furthermore, before what I shall too easily term "meaning" can be negotiated in the reading of *kanbun*, it is necessary to supplement the written text with Japanese grammatical particles, agglutinative inflections, and "conjugations." Thus, in itself, any text written in *kanbun* can never be conflated with the presence of a unitary authorial voice; indeed, the voice is always at once a displacement of, and supplement to, the written text. Furthermore, it is the Preface dated 1935 that should be written in modern Japanese, and the text proper, so called, that should be written in *kanbun*. Finally, the Preface situates Terukatsu's secret history within a series, or indeed a tradition, of *perverse*—that is to say, displaced and supplementary—sexuality: sadism, fetishism, homosexuality, sexualities that are construed to be mere imitations of what are always already constituted for us as the normal courses of desire. And so, to sign the Preface "Setsuyō gyōfu shiki" (*setsu*, both displacement *and* supplementarity; *yō* [Ch.: *yang*], the phallus; *gyōfu*, fisherman), a signature that supposedly guarantees the presence of the author to his readers, renders the Preface a parody of parody. In a series of deceptive stagings or framings, then, the author (but where is he?) recedes into otherness *from* the reader, revealing the scene of intersubjective recognition to be a specular trompe l'oeil.

The last sentences of the Preface ostensibly address the reader of the text directly, asking us not to dismiss the *Secret History* as an ill-conceived absurdity; we are enjoined, that is to say, to maintain a strict epistemological separation between the space of literature and the proper place of historiography. Yet insofar as we have already been alerted to the parodic nature of the text, it is impossible *not* to register the conjunction of "literary fiction" and historiographical representation. Is this conjunction merely a more or less straightforward matter of fiction, so called, being an entertaining parody of the high seriousness of historiography? Is fiction merely a displacement of, and supplement to, an altogether sober scholarship? Is fiction therefore in itself and as such essentially *perverse*, a perversion of the heroic monuments of history? Is the perversity of "erotic, grotesque literature"—*ero-guro bun*—no more than a distortion, albeit ironic, of the true, the straight, and the erect? Is the space of fiction therefore merely the "outside" of the authentic place, not only of historiography, but of what historiography invokes as "History itself"?

Or is it rather that fiction is the *truth* of history precisely because, in its very perversity, "literature," and the literature that is in all historiography, is both the displacement of and supplement to historiography proper and of "History itself"? In other words, that displacement and supplementarity, both unthinkable except as effects of the event of castration that is the advent of historicity (and that first and foremost displace and supplement the putative originality of that event), both intolerable obstacles to the achievement of identity, both unconscionable interferences in the accomplishment of intersubjective recognition and communication, and both anathema to historians who go straight to the point, are, as the truth of the lie of a feigned deception, as the dissemination that precedes origin, and as the essential dissembling of every resemblance, the phallus of history—that which is what it is only because, *as* truth, it is always missing, absent, undisclosed? So that when Tanizaki writes at the end of *In Praise of Shadows*, an elegy for the loss of a material culture, that it is only literature that can be the last refuge of nostalgia, has he already marked nostalgia as neither the mere reminiscence of plenitude nor even the acceptance of the loss of plenitude, but as the recognition that that plenitude was always already "lost"?[81] And that every recuperation of the plenitude of "Japanese culture"—and of "Japanese culture" as ontological plenitude—is the recuperation of an ontological plenitude that never was? The situation in Tanizaki is, I think, necessarily ambiguous, and because Tanizaki was never merely an ironist, must remain so—we owe him the acknowledgment of that ambiguity.

CHAPTER 7

The Death of Michel Foucault

It will be necessary to resist the tendency to render easy that
which cannot become easy without being distorted.

—Antonio Gramsci, *Selections from the Prison Notebooks*

The answer is the question's misfortune, its adversity.

—Maurice Blanchot, *The Infinite Conversation*

Suppose that it were still possible to think in relation to a certain figure, no less Imaginary than any other certainly, of Michel
Foucault. More precisely, suppose that it were still possible to think
what is at stake in thinking of a certain figure designated Michel
Foucault. Suppose that that would be to think of a Foucault who
was also something other than the thinker who apparently wrote
about nothing but pale male Europeans, a Foucault whom Jean
Baudrillard could never forget because he never read this Foucault,
a Foucault whose radicality has been eclipsed in the very invocation of a positivist Foucault by those who, curiously, seek the authority of their discourse in that very invocation, a Foucault who is
avoided precisely in the commitment of a questioning to hegemonic
contestation. Suppose that it were possible to think what might be
at stake in reading Foucault against Foucault, in reading Foucault
before he became, as H. D. Harootunian says, big business. Suppose, therefore, that it were possible to think about the figure of
Foucault as a series of questions about the very possibility of questioning, embarked upon what Blanchot called "research," where it
might be acknowledged that the only community we might achieve

is a community of the question, the question of the possibility of community. Which is to suppose that it would be possible to think what is at stake in thinking the figure of a *queer* Foucault.

Suppose further that it were possible to think the figure of a Foucault so radical as to break with Deleuze precisely on the question of desire, who rejected desire as the ontological limit, the Foucault who therefore identified individuals as the "pseudopodia of sexuality." Suppose that it were thereby possible to think what is at stake in the figure of a Foucault who could think power not only in its institutional inscriptions—both institution as inscription and inscription as institution—but also as the excess or surplus of institutionality and inscription altogether, a Foucault for whom power designated the radical impossibility of any grounding, thus enabling us to notice the illegal ground of all legality, the radically anarchic ground of all sociality, the groundlessness that is the ground of the political as such. Here would be a Foucault who taught us a reading of Nietzsche and Bataille, Blanchot's Foucault, a Foucault who would have understood Nishida's repeated claim that the ground and instauration of language lay in command and response, in the radical unjustifiability of Symbolic order as such, and therefore that the term "culture" names a separation that would be an originary separation from something other than "nature." Suppose, therefore, that it were possible to think the figure of a Foucault so radical as to be able to think an entire historical Imaginary predicated on the recognition that what "modernity" designates as madness is the absence of work, the radically *désoeuvrée*, and that the absence of work is the ground—as historicity, materiality, the Kantian manifold, the anarchic, in a word, power—of the logos, the Law, of culture, of what passes for civilization; a ground that can be glimpsed, beyond the representations that occlude it, at Dachau, Hiroshima, and Nagasaki, in the Gulag, in Cambodia and Vietnam, in the AIDS pandemic. Et cetera, most certainly et cetera.

Such would be to suppose that it were possible to turn to the figure of an uncompromising and intransigent Foucault, a Foucault whose *travail*, including that of his *oeuvre*, always suggested the possibility of an intervention rather than a hegemonic contestation, the

Foucault of a more than philosophical anarchism, who through the parodic refiguration of the historical Imaginary disclosed the impossible ground of that impossible object the political. Supposing all of this, and not just the sexy bits, would be to read the figure of the *queer* Foucault. Just suppose. Supposing *that*, where could we be?

Toward a Politics of Inconsolable Perversity

I have thus far attempted to attend to the necessary and radical insufficiency of thought to its objects, of thinking to that which it thinks it thinks when it thinks its thinking. In other words, I have tried to move toward a thinking of whatever it is that might be at stake *in positing* the necessary and radical insufficiency of thought to its objects, a thinking of what might be at stake in thinking the unthinkability of that which is strictly speaking unthinkable. It has been determinative for my attempt to make an approach to this question (an approach innumerable others have made before me) to try to think that insufficiency, not in the abstract generality of what can be thought, but in the specificity—or, indeed, singularities—of an irrecusable existential exigency; that is to say, as the non-negotiable demand upon thinking imposed by the events of 6 and 9 August 1945 (by the "objects" designated by the anonyms "Hiroshima" and "Nagasaki"), and by the AIDS pandemic. As objects of and for consciousness, "Hiroshima" and "Nagasaki" and "AIDS" are most certainly discursively constituted; yet there is that which is the unavoidable occasion of their discursive constitutions, and that makes of those discursive constitutions the thought of the force of existentiality. This is not to attempt to return in a nostalgic project to a putatively prediscursive uninscribed Real; rather, it is an attempt to approach the thought of the Real in its essential and radical historicity. I mean to say that to think the insufficiency or limit of thought in the rigorous specificity and singularity of that which it attempts to think is necessarily to attempt to think historically, both to think what thought attempts to think in *and as* its historicity, *and* to think the *thinking* of what thought attempts to think in *its* historicity as well. To think "Hiroshima," "Nagasaki," or "AIDS" in and as their nontranscendence is necessarily, by virtue of the exigency of their very existentiality, to think the nontranscendence— the limit, finitude, historicity—of any thinking about "Hiroshima," "Nagasaki," or "AIDS." It is this that has been determinative for my attempt to read Takenishi, Ōta, and Wojnarowicz.

Well, brave words, these; but if they are to be something other, even something more, than a presumptively salutary propaedeutic humiliation, a kind of proleptic catharsis or consolation, then they must register *for us*—and *now*—as something other, something more, than the transcendental insights of a contemplative passivity, as something other, something more, than an explanation or interpretation of the world. If the thought of the historicity of thought is not a rigorous praxis that calls everything, including its own possibility, into question, if it does not thereby submit it to a profound disruption, if it remains possible to continue to speak and to think in and as the reasonability of the sweet voice of reason, then everything that thinking has been, or might be, is nothing. If thinking accepts the "practical" constraints of its institution and institutions, then thought is nothing more than the administration, or policing, of its disciplines; and in that case, we shall have not even begun to think what it is imperative to think in this time of AIDS.

This final chapter is therefore neither a conclusion, nor a meditation on the impossibility of concluding. Rather, in reading certain fragments by Sue Golding (which will be a fragmentary reading), I want to try to pursue questions broached by Takenishi, Ōta, and Wojnarowicz in at least inchoate forms earlier in this investigation.[82] In what is perhaps its most general formulation, it is a question of the possibility of a praxis or various praxes oriented toward maintaining or bringing into being the possibility for politicality altogether, from within the prehistory of the political, a time when the very possibility of politicality as such is seemingly increasingly foreclosed. It is a question, therefore, not of a movement, faction, or party that would enter into a power struggle for hegemony over a totality (movements and parties that we know have only served to strengthen the foreclosure of the political: every revolution of our time has only reinforced the state-form as such, as Antonio Negri has reminded us). Rather, it is a question of molecular struggles, brushfires that illuminate, however briefly and however dimly, a "political" landscape against which the fulguration of a general revolutionary conflagration in the Jacobin Imaginary appears as nostalgic fantasy.

More specifically, however, it is a matter of the praxis of poiesis, of what it is we do in making whatever it is we make. It is a matter, therefore, of the tracing of a perverse nomadic itinerary, of staging, of the parodic, of play, of what Deborah Britzman calls "strange methods," which might disrupt, not only the instituted (and often enough institutionalized) normativities of what Wojnarowicz called the preinvented world, but also the very expectation of normativity altogether; it is a matter, therefore, of the perverse play of strange methods, which disclose the fundamental contingency of any possible normativity. It is, therefore, a matter of the praxis of poiesis as an erotics, an erotics of thinking, a political intervention sustained or justified by nothing save its own audacity, sovereignty or, as Sue Golding says, curiosity.

It is, therefore, a matter of whether it is possible even to pose the question of the ethical, for thinking the thought of the ethical. The question of the ethical comes to us, first and last, from beyond any possible epistemological horizon as a scream of abject, sovereign terror; it is indeed the call of a silent curse, which calls us and condemns us to a certain attention to an inassimilable singularity. The call of the ethical, the thought of the ethical, the thought that there is, or at least might be, an ethicality, is in its essence cruel, the very cruelty of thought itself. The thought of the ethical is the wound of trauma, the edge, the cut, the slash of the nontranscendence of the world, confronted with which we are bound to an impossibility of language that is no mere silence, and that is the only locus from which any language, any *signifiance*, any thought can possibly issue.

I read Golding on the relation of praxis and poiesis, as well as the praxis of her poiesis, imperatively to be grounded in, to be engaged by, to be called forth by, the ultimately unspeakable destitution that is the originary historicity of our being-in-common. It is in the first instance, that is to say, at the level of what would once have been called that of phenomenological experience, a matter of the punctuality of an attention to the finitude of whatever singularity, an attention to the punctuation of the deaths of the irreplaceable (but, as denizens of Agamben's Badaliya, substitutable) others: David, Lorne, Michael, Ricky, Danny, Andrew, Teddy, Sam, Tessa Boffin. No need, of course, to ask after the causes of these deaths, for they all died (whatever may have been the "motives" for Boffin's suicide) of "AIDS-related causes"; in the time of AIDS, we all live and die "in AIDS" (as one is said to live and die "in religion"), whether or not we die "of AIDS."

Consider, then, the address book (and the address book within "The Address Book"), the material exoskeletal articulation of a sociality, the grid of a set of geographical and technological coordinates that specifies and situates the multiple and constantly shifting foci of an attention to what is thereby never a sociality-in-general. The address book situates the other as the place of a possible address, the destination of an interpellation, the essentially fragile, tenuous, and contingent possibility of a relationality. The address book situates others in the citation of the propriety of the name, it locates the possibility of relation according to the protocols of the proper name, the singular predicate. But precisely in situating an other within a geographical, technological system that would constitute the possibility for relation, the errancy of a destination, the absence of response to an interpellation, the guarantee that others will be out of place, becomes possible. The address book, then, is at once the index of relation, of nonrelation, of the relation of nonrelation. It is in this respect then that "each name's inscription" is "too extreme" (AB, 173), unbearable in the inescapability of its destitution; the address book is the register in which the death of the friend is inscribed *en souffrance*, both the suspension of a punctuation and a suffering.

And, given that "the passage from the land of the un-deadness to some other shore is tricky indeed" (AB, 168), for "people in our condition" in this interminable time of AIDS, the decision to buy a new address book (the old bearing a too nearly unbearable resem-

blance to a necrology), as well as the rituals of its selection and purchase, are matters of the very greatest "delicacy," requiring the most
rigorous discipline, the most punctual attention. This disciplined,
punctual—in a word, historical—attention to the rituals of the
Book, must be marked by and as a rigorous attention to that of
which the Book is at once index and trace; but also that to which
the Book is a guide, a passage: in other words, "sociality" in the
unsublatability of its material (non-)relating relations. So it will be a
matter of attention to the materiality (the palpable relation to the
flesh, the skin, the sense of smell; even, although this flirts with abstraction, to the eye and the ear) of the Book, the ritual and its necessary accoutrements. The Book itself, of course, will have to be
black leather, discreet and severe, but "not without its smells, its
textures and its raunch" (AB, 168); on this historical, ritual excursion, one's comportment in the world—the praxis of a poiesis—
must be "utterly focused," a focus, an attention that will be expressed in the exactness of a sartorial severity, the precision of the
haircut. But this ritual attention to the historicity of a passage would
be merely a mortuary obsession were it inattentive to the pleasures,
pains, the pleasures of pain, the passages, the improbabilities, the
dangers, the contingencies, the *ekstases*, the tenuousness, the strangeness, the risks, and "that special kind of nakedness, so required of
each and every one of us" (AB, 168) of the erotic, the social.

Thus the slow soak in the hot baths to remind one, as the
body's afterburn, of "debauched pleasures" and "succulent pains";
the dildo or scarf worn next the skin "so as to call up the tongue of
S—— or maybe the hands of J——, sweeping gently but urgently
against my skin" (AB, 168); the pair of engraved silver tit clamps;
the gum wrapper inscribed with a poem from an old whore. A certain psychology would undoubtedly begin to speak disparagingly
of the fetish and of obsessional neurosis. Whatever. Here, rather let
us say that such material practices, such usages, such implements
are not merely mementos of the erotic (for it is not a symbolism
that is at stake here), but are *erotically* mementos of the erotic, of
erotic sociality; they are practices, usages, and implements that are,
even as they stand for or in the place of, the essential historicity or

impermanence of the social. Not merely memento mori, they nevertheless are indices of (even while they *are* in and as their being what and as they are) what is at stake in that which has been irrevocably lost. So something other than mourning or melancholia, something other than their alternation is at stake in the necessity of the Book. It is neither a matter of straightforward mourning, which would restore the ego to its historicist propriety, nor of the abjection of melancholia.

The narrative of the ritual of the address book is punctuated by an excursion—occasioned by the audacity, the sovereignty of "a craving directed only and always toward transforming forever (or at least for a few hours) a world without cunning or the pleasure of its dare" (AB, 169)—into Sodom, the city that promises the intimacy of "that strange hospitality so conspicuous to anyone on the prowl" (AB, 169), the city of the nomadic stranger to the *domus*, the city of that punctual attention that is cruising, the city that is outside the work and reason of the domestic community, the city outside the Law, the city of David Wojnarowicz, a city named both Sodom and Badaliya, the city of the outlaw, the city of an originary homelessness, in a word: home. But this Sodom is the site of a periodic apocalypse, for existing only in, and as, the interstices of geopolitical community, its inhabitants are periodically, albeit irregularly, subjected to police raids, demonstrations—as if they were needed—of the tenuous fragility of all sociality. Witness to all nine hundred moments of one such raid, the narrator rages against its horrors (a rage that is also a rage against the ravages of AIDS [PB, 30–31]), "until the I of me was reduced to a stunned and sickly silence" (AB, 170). An old whore recalls her to a consideration of Lot's Wife, "poor LW" (172), who too was witness to the annihilation of her people, for which, of course, she was transformed into a pillar of salt.

"For the blinding sight of the deep flash when the living goes to dead—the very transformation of Sodom and Gomorrah into the past tense of total annihilation—was precisely 'history', now; her history-now; exactly her memory, and, as such, it set the boundary over which she could not possibly leap." LW, then, is ossified precisely because she could not "attempt to sustain a present or future life endlessly rooted in the land of the dead. That would condemn any 'survivor' to a tearful emptiness so profound as to become no life at all." But the problem here is no mere melancholia, "For to re-live forever the very instant of that memory—the very instant of a life gone by . . . would always-already dry us right up— embodying the pristine absence of the future in the un-deadness of our gaze" (AB, 172). LW cannot, no more than we, no more than Takenishi, Ōta, or Wojnarowicz, no more, if to comes to that, than Benjamin's Angelus Novus, transcend the boundary of the limit-situation. Let us return LW and the Angelus Novus to their respective theologies; for us, it is neither the consolations of the historicizing work of mourning, nor the salty transfixed gaze of a melancholy monument. It is a certain audacity, a certain sovereignty, a certain perversity, "in the face of—rather than in spite of—all the mad pleasures and damnations and decay" that "begins with taking the memories of them: ALIVE; by carrying those memory figments forward and as close to the body parts as possible, playing with them, re-inventing them and . . . of 'never looking back'" (AB, 172–73). This is the "historical consciousness," then, of an awareness of the radical destitution of being in its historicity, which refuses either to occlude that destitution in historicization *or* to take up residence in the necropolis of the Imaginary. This double refusal therefore suggests an essential instability in the binary opposition of presence to absence; for it is a question of ghosts and angels. At the conclusion of her remarks at Tessa Boffin's funeral, Golding cites Boffin citing Rilke:

> But the living are wrong
> in the sharp
> distinctions they make.
>
> Angels, it seems,
> don't always know
> if they're moving among
> the living or the dead. (PB, 34)

It is not that there is no difference between life and death, as if in some consolatory gesture one could reverse the "no-going-back of life" (PB, 34). Rather, it suggests that it is in the audacity (or sovereignty) of the practice of a certain poiesis, constituted as a kind of kleptomania-cum-bricolage in the reinvention of pleasure and its instruments, in play, in ontological parapraxes, that the recognition of destitution becomes the condition of possibility for "history" as a movement toward futurity as difference. Thus, the address book and its attendant material rituals together become a poiesis, a making, that constitutes a punctual attention to apocalyptic destitution, but also and *thereby* to the impossibility of containment that is the social.

What was the occasion of LW's fatal nostalgia, other than sheer perversity; or rather, what is the perversity of that nostalgia? What surge of life in its sensuousness, in its sensuality, in its palpable vitality did LW (according to Sue Golding) regret so much as to sacrifice herself to the eternal contemplation of its extermination? In what does the impossibility-of-containment consist as to be the impossible (because evanescent) object for Golding's punctual attention? What would be the being-in-common of "buddies in bad times"?

We might begin to think an approach to these questions first of all in terms of Sue Golding's rhetorical address, and attend to the *domina's* interpellation by which we are called to readership, to attention, to the putative community constituted in the ways in which every text posits its intelligibility. The question is, *what* intelligibility is being presumed? Golding makes a gesture, which is surely not entirely a feint, an irony, to the reader for whom the possibility of intelligibility and sense is unquestionably always already there: "I will be quite frank with you," she promises in the address of "The Address Book" (AB, 168); a free and open exchange of views among folks who, surely, must be able to understand each other is without a doubt what we can expect from such an engaging author. And Golding does not disappoint. After a precise and loving description of the tit clamps, which will accompany her in the event of buying the Book, she assures us in a one-line paragraph that she and her reader constitute a community: "You know precisely what I mean" (AB, 169). Or again, dressed for a predatory foray in

Sodom, she notes, as part of her accoutrement, "the usual assort-
ment of toys—like hand-cuffs and rope (you know, things like that)"
(SM, 161). Or yet again, although she expresses regret that the
reader might be disappointed that she will not offer a "primer" on
"perverse behaviour" (SM, 162–63), she is confident that we too
have been exasperated by questions as to the whys and wherefores of
our being and behavior (SM, 164). Every reader, surely, is an acknowledged virtuoso with the tit clamps, the rope, the cuffs, and
has been irritated by the stupidity of those imbecile uncompre-
hending others. What I suggest, at the risk of underscoring the obvious and spoiling the fun, is that Golding's rhetorical address stages,
parodically to be sure, the recognition scene of an intersubjective
interpretative community within which intelligibility and sense are
precisely what goes without saying. For those of us for whom tit
clamps, cuffs, rope, and so on are indeed among the instruments of
play, the assurance of mutual understanding would be quite beside
the point; to suggest that something goes without saying can only
mean that it does in fact need saying. In any case, the virtually
preternatural solidarity of a community constituted in the intersubjective recognition of a shared intelligibility is being shaken here;
the reader can no longer situate herself and/or himself securely outside the field of the perverse. The point is driven home, perhaps,
when Golding suggests a quite specific perversity to intellectual clar-
ity: "And because I want to torture you ever so slightly, or, to put it
somewhat differently, because I want to make sure that this point
is clear" (SM, 164), she will turn to—Wittgenstein. The reader, recognized as one who, not without reason, knows something about
perversion, will have an increasingly difficult time, if such is his
and/or her bent, in contemplating the social as anything other than
a certain impossibility of containment. Sue Golding's address prohibits disavowal.

Golding is quite explicit on the point: "If what you want is to
'oooh' and 'aaah' from the other side, with your upturned noses
pressed against the *supposed* boundary between us, then: go away!"
(PB, 28). The full force of the thought of the social as noncontainment (or as Agamben's "unbinding") in Golding's rhetorical address

arrives as the next paragraph: "Let's face it: we're all in this together, oh gentle reader; and no one—and that includes you and me, both —gets out of here, alive" (PB, 28). Our sociality, our historicity— which is to say: our very existentiality *as* the equiprimordiality of our historicity and sociality—are therefore, and the point is not as obvious as it may sound, unavoidable. It is the material *inescapability* of our nontranscendence that must be taken to be the ground of our being-in-common, rather than any ontologically given essential similitude, whether that similitude be constituted as "identity" or "behavior." It is this inescapable vulnerability or destitution of a certain materiality—the body of this death, with the perversity of its pleasures, the succulence of its pains-that is the ground of the noncontainment, the nonreserve, that is our being-in-common. The referent of any "we," whether explicitly rhetorical or with ostensive reference, is necessarily and forever indeterminate; neither an indiscriminate holism nor the secure separation of the particular, the sociality of the we is that indeterminacy itself: "Dear, dear reader: how to begin to tell our story, without exploding into a million disconnected pieces or melting into one big globular humanistic blob? . . . If we cut ourselves, do we not bleed?" (PB, 29). Y su sangre ya viene cantando. Thus:

> So listen, please, oh kind and gentle reader! Do not turn your back on us. It is not just a Daddy who is dying! It is our brothers who are dying! It is, in fact, a whole people who is dying! . . . You cannot and will not divide us from each other: we are all in this together, fighting as we must so do, as this Death keeps coming after us, and after us, and after us. And it keeps on coming after us, even when it's not. (PB, 31)

Y su sangre ya viene cantando . . .

Nonreserve, indeterminacy, sociality: these are not predicates, attributes, or qualities that would adhere to or inhere in an object, "society," for example. They are, rather, being-in-common itself. The question of the social is therefore not a matter of a dialectic of universal and particular; it is not a question of the *identity* of the particular or the identities of multiple particularities in relation to one another; for, however complex the sophistications of such relations, the particular is, as the particular *of the universal*, nothing but a (negative) element of universality as such, the particular as the (negative) element that expresses the universal. The social is therefore not the fate or destiny of particularities. It is nevertheless a certain "toward-which," a "that-toward-which" that is neither telos nor destination; perhaps, however, a *lure*. Sociality can then only be thought, perversely, as the direction (and never the destination) of a certain movement, a certain precipitation, a "that-toward-which" a certain curiosity (yellow, blue, pink: whatever), a certain "interested intuition" *moves*. It might well be, then, that in Golding this nonreserve, indeterminacy, noncontainment (i.e., "the social"), *is* the call ("So listen, please, oh kind and gentle reader!"). I shall return to this, for how could one not?

If sociality is a "that-toward-which" that is a movement rather than a destination, if sociality is always "actualized" or "realized" in and as that very movement but never as a fully constituted object (that is also to say, never the actualization or realization of a possibility, for the possibility only appears as the realization or actualization of the movement), then the movement of realizing or actualizing sociality is the praxis of a poiesis, first and last erotic. That sociality, in its reductions to "society," "culture" or the "human," is effected by means of poiesis is of course no new insight. Poiesis has long been thought as that which realizes the object (a work of art, language, society, state, world, self, identity, the domus, the Law, culture, for example) as the result produced by an always already fully accomplished subjectivity (or a subjectivity that will be accomplished in and through poiesis) working upon raw materials (e.g., a world) according to rules that are the articulation of a technology grounded in a knowledge of the logos. And of course the dialectical sophistications of this narrative (introduced, for example—but what an example—by Marx) undoubtedly nuance the narrative in fundamentally important ways. But what has always been in question is a relation between a subjectivity that can at least possibly be accomplished as identity, and the regularities of a *technē* grounded in the logos. Poiesis, and the objects that are its effects, have together been subjected to judgment according to the terms of this relation. Crudely, a good person does the right thing, motives and morality, the why and the how and the what. In any case, what is considered essential is the depth of an interiority (being) and the *ground* of a technique; the surface, that is to say, necessarily conceals an authentic depth, the knowledge of which lends authority to judgment, and makes the thought of poiesis central to our intellectual police and to the polity of the philosopher-cop.

But this logic introduces what Golding calls the "Trojan Horse Dilemma," in which the assumption of that which is proved is embedded in the given, what a less audacious scholastic logic would call a *petitio principii* (SM, 163–65). Neither the "experience" of a subject to and as its identity nor "some overall objective Truth" to ground the truth can assure us of a knowledge of the rules of the game. Here, Golding turns to reflect on Wittgenstein in order to think the regularities of the rule in and through the exercise of the technique within which alone the rule exists. This is "a route, a mapping, an impossible geography—impossible not because it does not exist, but because *it exists and does not exist exactly at the same time*" (SM, 166). In other words, to offer a perhaps rather reductive translation, the rule exists as the always already there of inscription (on and as "bodies," for example); at the same time, the rule exists nowhere outside the practice or technique that is the rule's articulation. The rule (ultimately of every poiesis) contradictorily preexists its application and is reinvented in each performance thereof, existing only in and as its application; one plays the game according to rules that are made only in the play of the game: a disjunct simultaneity.

To pursue our translation of Golding a bit further. The prototype for this poiesis in which the ground is not a depth but a surface might, for example, be a musical performance or dance. In both cases, there is an itinerary, a mapping, as either a score or a choreography, and in that sense the "work" exists qua "work of art" prior to, or outside of, its actualization, as an accomplished, completed object. Yet at the same time, the music or dance "exists" *only* in the essential incompletion of its actualization, in the movement that is the surplus of its prior inscription as object. Indeed, as "prior" object, the score or choreography is the trace of the poiesis that is its supplement. The object exists, certainly, but it is the residue or trace of the poiesis that is necessarily always in excess of its objectivity (as *Gegenstandlichkeit*). As the object of a performativity, the object is always a temporalized object, a heard rather than a seen object. The object resides in the *essential* incompletion or unaccomplishment that *is* its poiesis—*and nowhere else*. Thus Golding:

> For there is no greater depth to a ground (itself fractured and multiple): *only the surface*, only the superficial interplay of, in this case, the sexual game; only, that is to say, the play of the game. The game as play: the technique of artifice and pleasure and tension and passion and limit and pain and threshold and lust and juices and sport, all pulling on, all pulling with, all pulling against the Joke—the erasing and presencing of the truth, the erasing and presencing of the game. (SM, 166)

Let me recapitulate what this thought of poiesis, a thought of instrumentality or usage as an erotics, would imply for any thought of the social. The social, that which is always necessarily in excess of a hypostatized object denominated "society," is itself a necessarily impossible object, impossible according to this logic of disjunct simultaneity in that it both does and does not exist qua object simultaneously. "The social," then, is the lure toward which poiesis moves but that is actualized or realized only as and in the play of that essentially ungraspable movement. This implies that a certain essential incompletion or unaccomplishment is sociality itself: sociality is the impossibility of accomplishing an authentic identity present to itself, the impossibility of grounding truth in the Truth. But this fact of the essential incompletion of sociality necessarily demands the recognition that sociality is always also at every moment fully accomplished, perfect (but *not* as object). Insofar as poiesis is movement itself, it is neither a degeneration of a previously accomplished form, nor the preparation or adumbration of an indefinitely deferred higher perfection: it is what it is in the suchness of "sociality as such." And this perfection "is" its very indeterminacy, "a story with no Morals" (SM, 167), as Golding says.

The social, therefore, can never be construed as a republic to be administered by the philosopher-cop, for its inhabitants lack the passports that would certify their being or nonbeing; its truth is, precisely, a nonrelation to Truth. The social is, without depth, the matter of surfaces, in the first instance of skin, the "one thing we have in common; to wit: our fantastical, drippy, colorful, tacky, often diseased, sometimes pimply, and otherwise bizarrely adorned, skin" (PB, 28). These surfaces, these skins, are in fact lamellae, surfaces and skins that are at once and therefore undecidably both inside and outside, including "the dark, the moist . . . the scented and the risk" (AB, 169) of asshole and cunt (SM, 167). The social is circumscribed by an impossible (i.e., both existing and nonexisting), infinitely fragile, evanescent, and effervescent geography, to which any sociological cartography is necessarily inadequate; a geography of relations that simultaneously appear and disappear in a net of "nodal points" (in "gossip," for example, "the 'that' of our sexual habits, conducts, manners" [SM, 167]—the "that" of our *signifiance*, that is to say). The social is an urban space, the city of Sodom: "A community, a queer (kind of) city (or better yet, cities) that, finally, not only privileges the Joke but has something to do with the cry: 'Freedom'" (SM, 161).

The social is the space of an originary ontological promiscuity, the "elsewhere" of a performative play "transforming forever (or at least for a few hours) a world without cunning or the pleasure of its dare" (AB, 169); the social becomes thereby a "spectacular space, a made-up, unreal, larger-than-life" space (SM, 161), a space constituted in and as the poiesis of the erotic performances of "dom, Master, bottom, whore-fem, butch, Daddy-boy, cruising, play, playmate and so on" (SM, 161). This is the space of "an aesthetic of existence as Existence," the "surface of the risk" (SM, 167). This poiesis becomes a staging, the operatic performance, not only of every presumptively discrete identity, but of identity as such. In staging multiple, frequently contradictory identities (which are something more and less that "just roles"), Tessa Boffin, in Sue Golding's recollection, staged (which means put at risk) the essential staginess, performativity, or poietic nature of identity itself (PB, 32–34), the performative parody of every Imaginary identification.

Consider, for example, the various scenes of rough sex and S/M. An extensive, albeit timid and embarrassed, psychological and psychoanalytical literature has analyzed S/M entirely in terms of its intersubjective dynamic, and therefore in terms of the confession of an innermost, ownmost guilty identity, a scene of confession that is a repetition of that to which the penitent patient, an impatient penitent, confesses.[83] Such analyses finally cannot but assume a strict correspondence, or in fact identity, of the "psychosexual" and political Imaginaries; every top becomes a candidate for the SS, every bottom the perfect subject of any authoritarian regime. The scene of S/M is thus identified as the scene of the master/slave dialectic: MS/SM. Among those of us for whom rough sex and S/M, in the multiplicity and proliferation of its practices and possibilities, are other than merely the object of and for a fascinated (disgusted) ethnology, sociology, or psychology, other than merely the *frisson* of the slightly naughty avant-garde, there have been those who have attempted to justify and legitimate S/M—in the name of, and as the expression of, a libertarianism; or as the relatively harmless, controlled acting out, or working out, cathartic in its essence, of a presumptively instinctual violent aggressivity; or in thinking the limit of pain as a spiritual liberation, for example. It would be irrelevant to the present argument to take issue with these various justifications, not because they are or are not persuasive, but because to do so would suggest that there is an essence to rough sex or S/M about which it is possible to argue. Nevertheless, I want to pursue another, less comforting, riskier, reading of the scene of rough sex or S/M, which refuses, not only the isomorphism of the psychosexual and political Imaginaries, but also the reduction of this proliferation of the multiple scenes of S/M to nothing but an intersubjective dynamic, whatever its sophistications. I want to argue that, at least for some of us, at least in some situations, and particularly in the texts of Sue Golding, the practices and possibilities of rough sex and S/M constitute a *poiesis without reserve*, a putting into play (*mettre en*

jeu) of the "body" in its material inescapability, as well as the putative identity of which the body is held to be at once the expression
and vehicle. Much is being refused here: identity, subjectivity, irony,
community construed as the self-containment of an essential similitude. Much is being affirmed here: the fundamental nonreserve of
play, the Joke, the parodic, invention (i.e., poiesis), the risk (of madness and death), in a word, pleasure. In these refusals and affirmations, what is being refused is the thought of any ultimate *justifiability*
of this poiesis without reserve; what is being affirmed (in a nonpositive affirmation) is the very unjustifiability of be-ing in its destitute historicity and sociality. And this affirmation is the audacity of
what Golding calls "curiosity," which I shall read as sovereignty, the
thought of which is the sole possibility for any thought of the ethical, for politicality as such.

So: the subject is bereft of her and/or his every ontological support; his and/or her Imaginary identifications, as well as every intersubjective recognition, are revealed to be essentially parodic, the
ludic performances of identities, bodies and recognitions, ontological drag: the Joke. "The Joke is not 'on us': it is us" (SM, 167);
"the Joke is neither real nor unreal; it is invention" (SM, 166). The
Joke, it might be said, it must be said, is originarily perverse; the
Joke is thereby a certain mettre en jeu, a putting into play of invention, the seductions of the "endlessly compelling attraction, the concrete infinity, of techne" (PFP, 3): an uncontainable poiesis entered
upon without reserve, *à corps perdu*. It is this poiesis or techne that is
itself the seductiveness of the social. This praxis of this poiesis or
techne undoubtedly results in an object, the "self," for example. But
this object, this self, can only be thought as the residual trace (nonetheless "real" for that) of the exposure to otherness (its excess), the
becoming other, that *is* its poietic invention (and that can never be
reduced to the immanent teleologies of *Bildung*)—the "self" is
nothing other than the alterities of the multiple, heterogeneous
"technologies of the self" that are its indeterminate "ecstatic" metamorphoses. And of course what would those technologies of the
self, this poiesis without reserve in Golding and Wojnarowicz, be,
other than the impossible geographies of the Wittgensteinian rule?

Now this implies a form of acephalic mastery, the mastery of an absolute vulnerability to *tuchē*. But before we proceed to this thought of the audacity of curiosity, of sovereignty, that is to say, two points bear emphasis.

First, as Golding succinctly puts it in a recent reading of Foucault, "The desiring subject is dead" (PFP, 5). If it is an infinite poiesis, the play of multiple technologies operating upon the surfaces of the fragmentary body, upon which rough sex and S/M open (if rough sex and S/M are, as the cut or wound that is not castration, the edge of the blade of a metamorphosis, the very seductiveness and seduction of that poiesis), if one surrenders, and in surrendering is given over to the sensuous and sensual play of an inescapable materiality, then it is not the emptiness that befalls a desiring subject (an identity) that is at stake, but a pleasure that would, as Foucault said, be "an event 'outside the subject' or on the edge of the subject, within something that is neither body nor soul, which is neither inside nor outside, in short a notion which is neither ascribed nor ascribable."[84] Thus, Foucault again:

> The idea that S&M is related to a deep violence, that S&M practice is a way of liberating this violence, this aggression, is stupid. We know very well that what all those people are doing is not aggressive; they are inventing new possibilities of pleasure with strange parts of their body—through the eroticisation of the body. I think it's a kind of creation, a creative enterprise. . . .
>   . . . One can say that S&M is the eroticisation of power, the eroticisation of strategic relations . . . the S&M game is very interesting because it is a strategic relation, because it is always fluid. Of course there are roles, but everyone knows very well that those roles can be reversed. Sometimes the scene begins with the master and slave, and at the end the slave has become the master. Or, even when the roles are stabilised, you know very well that it is always a game: either the rules are transgressed, or there is an agreement, either explicit or tacit, that makes them aware of certain boundaries. This strategic game as a source of bodily pleasure is very interesting.[85]

In various of its poietic practices, S/M most certainly stages the scenes of intersubjectivity, including its recognitions. But, precisely because it is a staging, and damn well knows it is a staging, a parodic simulacrum, it knows just as well that *every* intersubjectivity is a staged performance. And it is precisely in knowing that it is a staging, and in the eroticization of power, that a reflection upon S/M might begin to think the dispersions and deployments, indeed the play, of power.

Second, and concomitantly, performative parody opens upon the possibility, however slight, for the "lesbian hermaphrodite's" survival in the impasses of the current conjuncture, the time of AIDS. In "James Dean: The Almost-Perfect Lesbian Hermaphrodite," Golding is concerned with a sexual imaginary that emerged during the 1980's, one image of a lesbian hermaphrodism, "James Dean with a clit" (JD, 50). Neither androgyny, sartorial genderfuck nor the putative referent of a bio-medical science, the image of the (sometimes "lesbian") female hermaphrodite as such is figured within the Imaginary of nineteenth-century medical discourse. For not only were "hermaphrodites" (at least those who did not repent their bodies and physiologies) in and as their essential excess necessarily sexually transgressive and subversive; it was also the case, Q.E.D., that "female sexual subversives [undoubtedly including every woman who did not regret the sexual pleasures of the body] must *ipso facto*, be hermaphrodites" (JD, 51). The hermaphroditic woman of the nineteenth century, that fascinating object for medical science, "dies an empty pathetic little death" (JD, 51); but she has a modern counterpart, "the 'virile girl,' the butch baby, full of attitude but not of scorn, lots of street smarts and a bit of muscle" (JD, 52). Most important, she is public, not only by virtue of being out of the closet and out *there*, but as the "orphan of a people's imaginary," as "a composite copy of a mass invention, a replica of our own societal icons, which are themselves never anything other than a public fiction. She is James Dean over and over again" (JD, 52). She is an "infinite copying," who parodically performs "James Dean" (himself a simulacrum) as the "defiant aesthetic of the erotic masculine shot through with the voluptuousness of the female sexual organs" (JD, 52). Or rather, she is James Dean relieved of a certain "slight imperfection," for she is "the proud owner of a vaginal hole and a carbide clit"; no longer the embodiment of a lack, she becomes "a signature for lesbianism itself" (JD, 52). It is precisely because in the perepeteia of her pleasures, in her affirmation of sexual possibilities and practices, she cannot be reduced to the figure of the tragic, that for the prude (lesbian or straight), she "can only be the pornographic filth in the age of AIDS, the frankenstein without a cause" (JD, 52).

Because the lesbian hermaphrodite (but not in her "being") affirms the sexual (hence erotic and social) play of a parodic performativity, because she puts into play without reserve, in her passionate perversity, a certain zero-degree *aisthēsis*, she is rendered abject in respect of "the prudish world." But at the same time, precisely "because she is the composite series of an infinite erotic fiction, a fractured playfulness of social icons copied over and over again," she can, with luck and audacity, evade—or at least forestall—the crucifixion of identity, the crucifixion that *is* identity. The only hope of survival lies in the risk of the dare, the perverse audacity—the sovereignty—of putting oneself, and one's self, in play, in the perverse poiesis of becoming, over and over again, "James Dean," of "doing" James Dean, of jamesdeaning, or indeed, of suegolding: "The Joke is not 'on us': it is us" (SM, 167).

Insofar as the thought of this audacity, this sovereignty, this curiosity in Golding is the singular "vanishing point" at which the thought of ethicality becomes possible, it is necessary to attempt to specify this sovereignty as rigorously as possible. Clearly, curiosity, audacity, and sovereignty cannot be thought as qualities or attributes predicated on an ego, a willing subject, or even a self; it is that which overtakes and passes through an existent, leaving whatever ego may have stood in its way in bloody scraps. Sovereignty in this respect is something of what was once called the daemonic or, a bit more recently, the drive (*Trieb*); it will be closer to a "beheaded rational master of self" (PFP, 4), an acephalic, directed autopoiesis. Let us say, quite simply, but obscurely, that sovereignty emerges in the interested intuition of the ecstatic fetish.

In "Curiosity," a paper as yet unpublished, Golding pursues a critique of any dialectics (the Hegelian being perhaps the most pertinent) in which negativity could only ever be the negation of a prior positivity, the identity of any singularity only a particularity established as the negation of its other, heterogeneity merely the dispersion, and therefore immanence, of totality in difference. She pursues this critique to think the possibility of an originary heterogeneity (i.e., a heterogeneity that would be something other than the fragmentation of a prior unity), a radical pluralism. She therefore invites us to imagine a cut as something other than the virgule that divides "the something from its other," and that

> no longer demarcates a site of departure (or arrival) with respect to any truth or certainty, dialectical or otherwise, and despite its fiction (or because of it), rewrites a truth. It is closer in description to a "forgotten" homeland, a bleeding land as it were, whose very landscapes circumscribe the nomadic dislocation of the neither/nor—the multiplicities of which are wholly unthinkable without a radical reinvention/remembering of space (as the de-de-negation) and of time (as its displaced movement). (C, 19)

Let us make a leap, not without its risk, and claim that what Golding has in mind here is the ultimately ungraspable historicity, or historical space, that is the indifferent ground of any difference, the very destitution of the exhaustion of predication, the contradictory being-in-common of whatever singularities. Or, as Golding argues in effect, the political as such *is* this originary heterogeneity, always already mapped in the impossible geography, the topology, of the paradoxical rule that both exists and does not exist; the political is therefore not a public space into which pre- or reconstituted private beings enter, but that from which, and as which, every articulation emerges. And this thought of a negative pluralism (the being-in-common of whatever singularities) is the unique condition of possibility for a praxis oriented toward a future substantially different from the present. This radical heterogeneity is not, therefore, the "Hobbesian nightmare," the landscape of an entropic despair envisioned by critics of "postmodernity," but that solely according to the thought of which the fiction of freedom can be figured in the (revolutionary) Imaginary, the only possibility for articulating freedom (as something other than the negation of unfreedom—"nature," for example) in praxis. It is for this reason that the "spectacular . . . made-up, unreal, larger-than-life" space of the queer city (or cities) "not only privileges the Joke but has something to do with the cry: 'Freedom'" (SM, 161).

Now the passage to this freedom, this sociality, will not be through the defiles of "the Truth or the Temporal or the Ethical or the Moral or the Dialectical," but, "at its most modest point," curiosity, the "ever-impossible journey 'to find out'" (C, 26). Curiosity, or interestedness, is thought, in the first instance, not so much as a quality or attribute of a being, but as the movement of the relation of nonrelation in the direction of the originary heterogeneity of whatever singularities, the erotic sensuousness of the infinitely various surfaces of what is. Curiosity is an interested intuition (or what Nishida Kitarō called "acting [or active] intuition" (*kōiteki chokkan*).[86] I may be curious, but there is that which arouses my curious imagination, which bestirs me from my dialectical slumbers into the poietic praxes of the play of heterogeneity. That which awakens me, that which attracts my curiosity, is not the impossible object of desire—nothing so profound, Golding would admonish—but an insignificant little something, a bare scrap of *signifiance*, a lure: the "ecstatic fetish." Here, the fetish is "ecstatic" in the sense we have seen Golding read in Foucault. The fetish, no "signifier of Death or of a failed Mourning or of a melancholia-writ-large-and-inescapable" (PFP, 7), "*is precisely and only—the multiple singularity of: itself*" (PFP, 8). The fetish is "an obsessional, virtual, metonymic surface. An unreal (but on the other hand, no less real), floating, magical, pleasure seeking surface, shot through with the absurdity of the cruel, of the dead, of the wronged. . . . A cyberspace of present tense passion, of perpetual movement going nowhere in particular, but going there with speed and agility and attentiveness to detail, nonetheless" (PFP, 9). The fetish, quite simply, is the vanishing point of materiality; the finite transcendence of the punctuation of what is; in Christopher Fynsk's phrase, the "bite of the Real"; the point at which predication is exhausted. The fetish, precisely in its materiality, is the provocation of a passionate, erotic intuition: "that it is there," in its

essential and necessary flight from the grasp of a being (or of being), is what precipitates the unjustifiable movement of the poietic
curiosity by which any I is overtaken. Thus:

> Its presence, like all presents, is simply impossible (here, there, and
> gone at the exact same instant); a virtual "to be," a mastery of the
> coming of masterliness. A radical mastery: being a perfectly imper-
> fect autonomous mastering, as de Sade would say, one without sub-
> mission to a fixed and totalized Other. It is rather a *virtual* mastery, a
> radically impure mastery—de-sanitized over and again on the slip-
> pery slope between and amongst the relation of self to self. (PFP, 9)

If the fetish is a scrap of nothing very much, which nevertheless
arouses the undead to the very movement of poiesis, then it cannot be what philosophers might call the sufficient cause of the play
of that poiesis. In other words, the movement of poiesis "toward"
the fetish, this passionate intuition of the fetish, is without ground,
unjustified. And it is this impossibility of grounding, this very unjustifiability of the erotic intuition of the fetish in flight, that *is* the
sovereignty of the praxis of poiesis. Just as "power" in Foucault indicates, among much else perhaps, the impossibility of grounding
the political (because the political as such is an originary heterogeneity), so, too, it is this sovereign perversity of poiesis that indicates the impossibility of grounding imagination in Truth, an impossibility Golding marks with the term "freedom." Now this sovereignty constitutes a mastery (albeit "virtual"), a control, even a
discipline (as in Foucault's technologies of the self); but, because
this sovereignty is grounded in neither identity nor Truth (because,
that is to say, this sovereignty is entirely unapologetic), because it
expresses no ontology, because it is anarchic, it marks the radical
contingency of every rule and every relation, the illegality of the
Law as such *and* the exceptional character, the fragility of every relation, the fact that every rule, every relation is sustained only by
the sovereignty of its enactment, its poiesis, the praxis of its poiesis.

Now it is this awareness of the artifices of sovereignty that
makes the thought of the ethical possible. It is only if we can imagine the sheer audacity of sovereign play, only if we can imagine that

what we do in making what we make is sustained by nothing but the sheer improbability of it all, the fact that it could be quite otherwise, that we can think the thought of the ethical. Which is to say that the question of the ethical is in itself a cruel question, a painful question, which always throws us into the limit-situation where the very possibility of speaking, of thought, is the most improbable of possibilities. For the ethical is the insistence of a demand, a call, a scream of abject terror, that comes to us from the sociality, the indeterminacy, the nonreserve, that is beyond every epistemological horizon. The ethicality of the ethical resides only in broaching the question of the ethical, and in the unremitting cruelty of a question that must be borne in the *askēsis* of an unbearable silence.

Reference Matter

Notes

1. John Greyson, *Zero Patience*, 100 min., Cinevista Video, 1993.

2. David Wojnarowicz, Untitled 1992, Gelatin-silver print and silk-screened text, 38" x 26". A reproduction may be found in *David Wojnarowicz: Brush Fires in the Social Landscape* (New York: Aperture, 1994), 83.

3. Michel Foucault, *The Archaeology of Knowledge*, trans. A. M. Sheridan Smith (New York: Harper & Row, 1972), 17.

4. There has been a widespread acknowledgment of the radical apocalyptic dimensions of the AIDS pandemic in various political actions (ACT UP, OutRage, AIDS Action Now, etc.), in the incorruptible intransigence of diverse video and performance artists such as John Greyson and Diamanda Galás, in film (such as the work of Derek Jarman), and in the statements and daily practices of People Living With AIDS, and so forth. But this has been an acknowledgment in which intellectuals, *as* intellectuals, have by and large refused to participate. Among the very few who have seriously begun to think what might be a stake for *thinking* with respect to the pandemic, Avital Ronell was one of the first, in 1983, to publish in English. See her essay "Queens of the Night," in *Finitude's Score: Essays for the End of the Millennium* (Lincoln: University of Nebraska Press, 1994), 41–61. See also Alexander García Düttmann, "What Will Have Been Said About AIDS: Some Remarks in Disorder," trans. Andrew Hewitt, *Public* 7 (1993): 95–114; Linda Singer, *Erotic Welfare: Sexual Theory and Politics in the Age of Epidemic*, ed. Judith Butler and Maureen MacGrogan (New York: Routledge, 1993); and Jacques Derrida with *Autrement*, "The Rhetoric of

Drugs: An Interview," trans. Michael Israel, *differences* 5, no. 1 (Spring 1993): 1–25.

5. For a journalist's account, valuable precisely because of the problematic nature of its representational strategies, see Randy Shilts, *And the Band Played On: Politics, People and the AIDS Epidemic* (New York: St. Martin's Press, 1987); for other, more ostensibly sober accounts, see Mirko D. Grmek, *History of AIDS: Emergence and Origin of a Modern Pandemic,* trans. Russell C. Maulitz and Jacalyn Duffin (Princeton: Princeton University Press, 1990); Barry D. Schoub, *AIDS and HIV in Perspective: A Guide to Understanding the Virus and its Consequences* (Cambridge, Eng.: Cambridge University Press, 1994); and, of course, Cindy Patton, *Inventing AIDS* (New York: Routledge, 1990), esp. 51–75.

6. It is interesting to note that in *AIDS: The Burden of History* (Berkeley: University of California Press, 1988), the editors, Elizabeth Fee and Daniel M. Fox, assumed that the categories of continuity and tradition of a normative historiography were entirely adequate to the object; by the time they edited *AIDS: The Making of a Chronic Disease* (Berkeley: University of California Press, 1992), they were considerably less convinced—only to find the "chronic" to be a concept adequate to its object. In a not entirely dissimilar strategy, Gilbert Herdt and Shirley Lindenbaum, editors of *The Time of AIDS: Social Analysis, Theory, and Method* (Newbury Park, Calif.: Sage Publications, 1992), suggest that "the disease of AIDS" is changing the ways in which the social sciences analyze "reality" (3), only to agree in conclusion that "a 'deconstructive' postmodern stance, which asserts that the world is imaginary, does not provide the appropriate forum" for any thinking about AIDS (328). As arrogant as it is moronic, this unconscionable refusal to think seriously nevertheless leads Herdt and Lindenbaum to the criminal consolation that "[w]e bear the burdens of AIDS better by knowing that we are contributing, in however small ways, to its ultimate defeat" (21). It is precisely the intellectual dishonesty of such feints that obviates any possibility for consequent thinking with regard to the pandemic.

7. In addition to Cindy Patton's *Inventing AIDS,* many of the essays in *Ecstatic Antibodies: Resisting the AIDS Mythology,* ed. Tessa Boffin and Sunil Gupta (London: Rivers Oram Press, 1990), pursue the question. See also the essays in *AIDS: Cultural Analysis, Cultural Activism,* ed. Douglas Crimp (Cambridge, Mass.: MIT Press, 1988), esp. Paula A. Treichler, "AIDS, Homophobia, and Biomedical Discourse: An Epidemic of Signification," 31–70. Also important are Simon Watney, *Policing Desire: Pornography, AIDS and the Media* (Minneapolis: University of Minnesota Press, 1987) and many

of Watney's essays collected in his recent *Practices of Freedom: Selected Writing on HIV/AIDS* (Durham, N.C.: Duke University Press, 1994).

8. Thus David McBride, in *From TB to AIDS: Epidemics Among Urban Blacks Since 1900* (Albany: State University of New York Press, 1991), concludes that "in the future, given the history and force of racial stratification in the United States, no Americans, regardless of color, will be able to approach the dynamics of racial discriminations and the AIDS epidemic as separable problems" (171). The pertinent literature is very large indeed, but I have found the following works to be particularly provocative: Paul Farmer, *AIDS and Accusation: Haiti and the Geography of Blame* (Berkeley: University of California Press, 1992); Panos Institute, *AIDS and the Third World* (Philadelphia: New Society Publishers, 1989); Renée Sabatier, *Blaming Others: Prejudice, Race and Worldwide AIDS* (Philadelphia: New Society Publishers, 1988); Richard Chirimuuta and Rosalind Chirimuuta, *AIDS, Africa and Racism*, rev. ed. (London: Free Association Books, 1989); Mehboob Dada, "Race and the AIDS Agenda," in *Ecstatic Antibodies*, ed. Boffin and Gupta, 85–95; Simon Watney, "Missionary Positions: AIDS, 'Africa,' and Race," in *Practices of Freedom*, 103–20; Cindy Patton, "Inventing 'African AIDS,'" in *Inventing AIDS*, 77–97; Paula A. Treichler, "AIDS and HIV Infection in the Third World: A First World Chronicle," in *AIDS: The Making of a Chronic Disease*, ed. Fee and Fox, 377–412; Diane Richardson, *Women and AIDS* (New York: Routledge, 1988); ACT UP / NY Women and AIDS Book Group, *Women, AIDS and Activism* (Boston: South End Press, 1990); *Working with Women and AIDS: Medical, Social and Counseling Issues*, ed. Judy Bury, Val Morrison, and Sheena McLachlan (New York: Tavistock/Routledge, 1992); and Cindy Patton, *Last Served?: Gendering the HIV Pandemic* (London: Taylor & Francis, 1994).

9. The actual extent of the pandemic is, of course, widely and vehemently disputed, but for some sense of the dimensions in which these questions need to be thought of, see *AIDS in the World*, ed. Jonathan Mann, Daniel J. M. Tarantola, and Thomas W. Netter (Cambridge, Mass.: Harvard University Press, 1992).

10. The discourse on "safer sex" is extensive. For serious introductions to pertinent discussions, see Singer, *Erotic Welfare*; Patton, *Inventing AIDS*, 25–49; Watney, *Policing Desire*; Watney, *Practices of Freedom*, 127–42; Edward King, *Safety in Numbers: Safer Sex and Gay Men* (New York: Routledge, 1993); Tessa Boffin, "Angelic Rebels: Lesbians and Safer Sex," in *Ecstatic Antibodies*, ed. Boffin and Gupta, 57–63; Douglas Crimp, "How to Have Promiscuity in an Epidemic," in *AIDS: Cultural Analysis, Cultural Activism*, ed. Crimp, 237–70; Simon Watney, "The Possibilities of Permuta-

tion: Pleasure, Proliferation, and the Politics of Gay Identity in the Age of AIDS," in *Fluid Exchanges: Artists and Critics in the AIDS Crisis*, ed. James Miller (Toronto: University of Toronto Press, 1992), 329–67; and John Greyson, "Still Searching," in *A Leap in the Dark: AIDS, Art and Contemporary Cultures*, ed. Allan Klusaček and Ken Morrison (Montreal: Véhicule Press, 1992), 85–95. Also important to these discussions, although not directly concerned with questions of AIDS and "safer sex," are Donna J. Haraway, *Simians, Cyborgs, and Women: The Reinvention of Nature* (New York: Routledge, 1991), 203–30; and Emily Martin, *Flexible Bodies: Tracking Immunity in American Culture from the Days of Polio to the Age of AIDS* (Boston: Beacon Press, 1994).

11. My thinking here is particularly indebted to the work of Nishida Kitarō. Virtually—and practically—all of that work is pertinent, but the preceding paragraphs rely in particular upon the later essays in *Mu no jikakuteki gentei*, in *Nishida Kitarō zenshū*, 2d ed., ed. Abe Yoshishige et al. (Tokyo: Iwanami, 1965–66) (hereafter cited as *NKz*), vol. 6.

12. Perhaps one of the most thoughtful mediations on AIDS, historicity, the historical Imaginary, and historiographical representation is John Greyson's "movie musical" *Zero Patience*.

13. See Andrea Liss, "Contours of Naming: The Identity Card Project and the Tower of Faces at the United States Holocaust Museum," *Public* 8 (1993): 108–34. Two readings of the AIDS quilt that I find very problematic, however, are Judy Elsley, "The Rhetoric of NAMES Project AIDS Quilt: Reading the Text(ile)," in *AIDS: The Literary Response*, ed. Emmanuel S. Nelson (New York: Twayne, 1992), 187–96; and Peter S. Hawkins, "Naming Names: The Art of Memory and the NAMES Project AIDS Quilt," *Critical Inquiry* 19, no. 4 (Summer 1993): 752–79.

14. The Denver Principles may be found in ACT UP / NY Women and AIDS Book Group, *Women, AIDS and Activism*, 239–40. On political funerals, see Watney, *Practices of Freedom*, 250–52; and Jack Ben-Levi, "From Euphoria to Sobriety, from Reverie to Reverence: David Wojnarowicz and the Scenes of AIDS Activism," *Public* 8 (1993): 138–59.

15. On the historicity that resists historicization absolutely, see Theodor W. Adorno, *Negative Dialectics*, trans. E. B. Ashton (New York: Continuum, 1983); Maurice Blanchot, *The Writing of the Disaster*, trans. Ann Smock (Lincoln: University of Nebraska Press, 1986); idem, *The Infinite Conversation*, trans. Susan Hanson (Minneapolis: University of Minnesota Press, 1993), esp. 83–281 on "The Limit Experience"; Jacques Derrida, *Cinders*, trans. and ed. Ned Lukacher (Lincoln: University of Nebraska Press, 1991); idem, *Aporias*, trans. Thomas Dutoit (Stanford: Stanford University Press, 1993); Shoshana Felman and Dori Laub, *Testimony: Crises of*

Witnessing in Literature, Psychoanalysis and Art (New York: Routledge, 1992); Julia Kristeva, *Powers of Horror: An Essay on Abjection*, trans. Leon S. Roudiez (New York: Columbia University Press, 1982); Dominick LaCapra, *Representing the Holocaust: History, Theory, Trauma* (Ithaca, N.Y.: Cornell University Press, 1994); Jean-François Lyotard, *The Differend: Phrases in Dispute*, trans. George Van Den Abbeele (Minneapolis: University of Minnesota Press, 1988); and Edith Wyschogrod, *Spirit in Ashes: Hegel, Heidegger and Man-Made Mass Death* (New Haven: Yale University Press, 1985). On historicization as a form of disavowal (*Verleugnung*), see Jean-Luc Nancy, "Our History," trans. Cynthia Chase, Richard Klein, and A. Mitchell Brown, *Diacritics* 20, no. 3 (1990): 97–115.

16. The chronicles of ACT UP, AIDS Action Now, OutRage, and similar groups have yet to be written; but for an introduction to some of the discursive and representational strategies of ACT UP / NY, see Douglas Crimp with Adam Rolston, *AIDS Demo Graphics* (Seattle: Bay Press, 1990); for many of the problems that ACT UP / NY has encountered in terms of its own political organization, particularly insofar as it was dominated largely by white, middle-class gay men, see Catherine Saalfield and Ray Navarro, "Shocking Pink Praxis: Race and Gender on the ACT-UP Front Lines," in *Inside Out: Lesbian Theories, Gay Theories* (New York: Routledge, 1991), ed. Diana Fuss, 341–69; cf. Douglas Crimp, "Right on, Girlfriend!" *Social Text* 33 (1992): 2–18. Also important, of course, are Larry Kramer, *Reports from the Holocaust: The Making of an AIDS Activist* (New York: St. Martin's Press, 1989); Sarah Schulman, *My American History: Lesbian and Gay Life During the Reagan/Bush Years* (New York: Routledge, 1994); and George M. Carter, *ACT UP, the AIDS War and Activism*, Open Magazine Pamphlet Series, no. 15, updated ed. (Westfield, N.J.: Open Magazine, 1992).

17. Few reflections on pedagogy, including much of what passes for a radical "critical" pedagogy, take up the question of the *possibility* of any pedagogy in the light of this absence of specularity in serious terms. The work of Deborah P. Britzman constitutes an almost singular exception. For an introduction to this work, see Britzman, "Is There a Queer Pedagogy? Or, Stop Reading Straight," *Educational Theory* 45, no. 2 (Spring 1995): 151–65.

18. The texts I have in mind include a series of lectures delivered at Kyoto Imperial University in 1938 under the title *Nihon bunka no mondai*, which may now be found in *NKz*, 14: 387–417 (an expanded version was published in 1941; the text is reprinted in *NKz*, 12: 275–394); his lecture to the Shōwa emperor in January 1941, *Goshinkō sōan: Rekishiteki tetsugaku ni tsuite* (*NKz*, 12: 267–72); and a series of essays first published as a supple-

ment to vol. 4 of the philosophical essays, which may now be found in *NKz*, 12: 397–434. The third of these, *Sekai shin chitsujō no genri*, was the address to the Kokukaku kenkyūkai (*NKz*, 12: 426–34).

19. The most concise readily available English-language introduction to Japanese government wartime propaganda and ideology is perhaps John W. Dower, *War Without Mercy: Race and Power in the Pacific War* (New York: Pantheon Books, 1986), 201–90.

20. *NKz*, 12: 416–19.

21. Ibid.: 271–72.

22. This articulation of "absolute contradictory self-identity" is quite central to the entire body of work of Nishida's last decade, as Nishida himself noted. But for a concise formulation, see the essay entitled, aptly enough, *Zettai mujunteki jikō dōitsu*, in *NKz*, 9: 147–222.

23. *NKz*, 12: 426–27.

24. Ibid.: 428–30.

25. Friedrich Meinecke, *Historism: The Rise of a New Historical Outlook*, trans. J. E. Anderson (London: Routledge & Kegan Paul, 1972).

26. Antonio Gramsci, *Selections from the Prison Notebooks*, trans. and ed. Quintin Hoare and Geoffrey Nowell Smith (New York: International Publishers, 1971), 465.

27. Ibid., 405–6.

28. For this thought of "communism" as the historico-social futurity that necessarily exceeds any objectification or conceptualization as "history" or "society," see Jean-Luc Nancy, *The Inoperative Community*, trans. Peter Connor et al., ed. Peter Connor (Minneapolis: University of Minnesota Press, 1991), 71–81; and Félix Guattari and Toni Negri, *Communists Like Us: New Spaces of Liberty, New Lines of Alliance*, trans. Michael Ryan (New York: Semiotext[e], 1990).

29. Antonio Negri, *The Politics of Subversion: A Manifesto for the Twenty-First Century*, trans. James Newell (Cambridge, Eng.: Polity Press, 1989), 170. Michael Hardt has pointed out to me that Negri is here actually citing the Marx of the *Eighteenth Brumaire* rereading the Marx of the *Theses on Feuerbach*.

30. On the seductions and impasses of apocalyptic thinking, see Jacques Derrida, "On a Newly Arisen Apocalyptic Tone in Philosophy," trans. John Leavey, Jr., in *Raising the Tone of Philosophy: Late Essays by Immanuel Kant, Transformative Critique by Jacques Derrida*, ed. Peter Fenves (Baltimore: Johns Hopkins University Press, 1993), 117–71; cf. Fenves's "Introduction: The Topicality of Tone," in the same volume, 1–48; with regard to Hiroshima, see Peter Schwenger and John Whittier Treat, "America's Hiroshima, Hiroshima's America," *Boundary 2* 21, no. 1 (Spring 1994):

233–53; with regard to AIDS, see Lee Edelman, *Homographesis: Essays in Gay Literary and Cultural Theory* (New York: Routledge, 1994), 79–117; Richard Dellamora, *Apocalyptic Overtures: Sexual Politics and the Sense of an Ending* (New Brunswick, N.J.: Rutgers University Press, 1994); and Michael Lynch, "Terrors of Resurrection 'by Eve Kosofsky Sedgwick,'" in *Confronting AIDS Through Literature: The Responsibilities of Representation*, ed. Judith Laurence Pastore (Urbana: University of Illinois Press, 1993), 79–83.

31. Takenishi Hiroko, "The Rite," trans. Eileen Kato, in *The Crazy Iris and Other Stories of the Atomic Aftermath*, ed. Kenzaburō Ōe (New York: Grove Press, 1985), 169–200; Ōta Yōko, *City of Corpses*, in *Hiroshima: Three Witnesses*, trans. and ed. Richard H. Minear (Princeton: Princeton University Press, 1990), 143–273. All citations are given parenthetically in the text.

32. Sigmund Freud, in Freud and Josef Breuer, *Studies in Hysteria*, in *The Standard Edition of the Complete Psychological Works of Sigmund Freud*, trans. and ed. James Strachey et al. (London: Hogarth Press & Institute of Psycho-Analysis, 1954–76 [hereafter cited as *SE*]), 2: 162.

33. Sigmund Freud, "Mourning and Melancholia," in *SE*, 14: 253.

34. Ibid., 246.

35. Ibid., 249. My emphasis.

36. In thinking about the work of mourning, I have, in addition to the classic Freudian texts, also found useful Julia Kristeva, *Black Sun: Depression and Melancholia*, trans. Leon S. Roudiez (New York: Columbia University Press, 1989); Laurence A. Rickels, *Aberrations of Mourning: Writing on German Crypts* (Detroit: Wayne State University Press, 1988). On mourning in relation to AIDS, see Douglas Crimp, "Mourning and Militancy," *October* 51 (Winter 1989): 3–18; Jeff Nunokawa, "'All the Sad Young Men': AIDS and the Work of Mourning," in *Inside/Out*, ed. Fuss, 311–23; and Tim Dean, "The Psychoanalysis of AIDS," *October* 63 (Winter 1993): 83–116.

37. Maurice Blanchot, *The Unavowable Community*, trans. Pierre Joris (Barrytown, N.Y.: Station Hill Press, 1988), 25.

38. Derrida, "Rhetoric of Drugs," 20.

39. Michel de Certeau, *The Writing of History*, trans. Tom Conley (New York: Columbia University Press, 1988), 56–113.

40. This is a thematics pursued, of course, in previously cited work; see Lyotard, *Differend*; Felman and Laub, *Testimony*; and LaCapra, *Representing the Holocaust*.

41. Blanchot, *Infinite Conversation*, 130–35.

42. Jean-François Lyotard, "*Domus* and the Megalopolis," in *The Inhu-

man: Reflections on Time, trans. Geoffrey Bennington and Rachel Bowlby (Stanford: Stanford University Press, 1991), 191–204.

43. I quote the term "finite transcendence" from Fynsk's introduction to *On Language and Relation* (Stanford: Stanford University Press, forthcoming). His *Heidegger: Thought and Historicity*, expanded ed. (Ithaca, N.Y.: Cornell University Press, 1993), constitutes, of course, a movement toward this thought of "finite transcendence."

44. Blanchot, *Infinite Conversation*, 3–10.

45. Or what Nishida called the "continuity of discontinuity" (*hirenzoku no renzoku*): see *Sekai no jikō dōitsu to renzoku* in *NKz*, 8: 7–106.

46. Sigmund Freud, *Beyond the Pleasure Principle*, in *SE*, 12: 12–13.

47. My considerations of the "corpse" rely very heavily upon Maurice Blanchot, "Two Versions of the Imaginary," in *The Gaze of Orpheus and Other Literary Essays*, trans. Lydia Davis, ed. P. Adams Sitney (Tarrytown, N.Y.: Station Hill Press, 1981), 79–89; and upon the two chapters on Blanchot in Christopher Fynsk, *On Language and Relation*.

48. For an introduction to this thematics, central to Nishida-philosophy, see *Basho*, in *Hataraku mono kara miru mono e*, in *NKz*, 4: 208–289.

49. Singer, *Erotic Welfare*, 31.

50. Lyotard, *The Inhuman*, 193.

51. Dennis J. Schmidt, *The Ubiquity of the Finite: Hegel, Heidegger and the Entitlements of Philosophy* (Cambridge, Mass.: MIT Press, 1988), 218.

52. I refer to remarks Asada Akira made on "cultural inoculation" and the AIDS pandemic at an informal meeting at the University of Chicago in March 1987. Subsequent discussions with Yukiko Hanawa have also helped me to think about the issues involved.

53. Negri, *Politics of Subversion*, 122–26, 191–99; see also Guattari and Negri, *Communists Like Us*.

54. Karatani Kojin, *The Origins of Modern Japanese Literature*, trans. Brett de Bary et al. (Durham, N.C.: Duke University Press, 1993), 11–44; cf. Lyotard, "Scapeland," in *The Inhuman*, 182–90.

55. As Lyotard writes, "Let us at least bear witness, and again, and for no-one, to thinking as disaster, nomadism, difference and redundancy. Let's write our graffiti since we can't engrave.—That seems to be a matter of real gravity. But still I say to myself: even the one who goes on bearing witness, and witness to what is condemned, it's that she isn't condemned, and that she survives the extermination of suffering. That she hasn't suffered enough, as when the suffering of having to inscribe what cannot be inscribed without a remainder is of itself the only grave witnessing. The witness of the wrongs and the suffering engendered by thinking's *différend* with what it does not manage to think, this witness, the writer, the megalopo-

lis is quite happy to have him or her, his or her witnessing may come in useful. Attested, suffering and the untameable are as if already destroyed. I mean that in witnessing, one also exterminates. The witness is a traitor" (*The Inhuman*, 203–4).

56. Paul Hallam, *The Book of Sodom* (London: Verso, 1993), 13–96.

57. David Wojnarowicz, *Close to the Knives: A Memoir of Disintegration* (New York: Random House, Vintage Books, 1991), 116–17. Hereafter cited parenthetically in the text as *CK*.

58. David Wojnarowicz, *Memories That Smell Like Gasoline* (San Francisco: Artspace Books, 1992), 59. Hereafter cited parenthetically in the text as *MSG*.

59. For a particularly mordant account of the test and the diagnosis, see David B. Feinberg, *Spontaneous Combustion* (New York: Penguin Books, 1991), 69–81.

60. Jacques Lacan, *The Seminar of Jacques Lacan*, ed. Jacques-Alain Miller, Book VII: *The Ethics of Psychoanalysis, 1959–1960*, trans. Dennis Porter (New York: Norton, 1992), 60.

61. Giorgio Agamben, *The Coming Community*, trans. Michael Hardt (Minneapolis: University of Minnesota Press, 1993), 38.

62. Barry Blinderman, ed., *David Wojnarowicz: Tongues of Flame* (Normal, Ill.: University Galleries of Illinois State University; New York: Distributed Art Publishers, 1990), 54.

63. In addition to work I have already cited by Douglas Crimp, Simon Watney, and David B. Feinberg, see Leo Bersani, "Is the Rectum a Grave?" in *AIDS: Cultural Analysis, Cultural Activism*, ed. Douglas Crimp, 197–222; Frank Browning, *The Culture of Desire: Paradox and Perversity in Gay Lives Today* (New York: Crown, 1993); Gary Indiana, *Horse Crazy* (New York: Plume, 1990); idem, *Gone Tomorrow* (New York: Pantheon Books, 1993); Samuel R. Delany, *The Mad Man* (New York: Masquerade Books, 1994). The list could be extended indefinitely to include videos by Marlon Riggs, such as *Tongues Untied*, and John Greyson, such as *Zero Patience*, and many others.

64. Herbert Marcuse, *Eros and Civilization: A Philosophical Inquiry into Freud* (Boston: Beacon Press, 1966); Guy Hocquenghem, *Homosexual Desire*, trans. Daniella Dangoor (London: Allison & Busby, 1978).

65. Jacques Lacan, *The Four Fundamental Concepts of Psycho-Analysis*, trans. Alan Sheridan, ed. Jacques-Alain Miller (New York: Norton, 1977), 276.

66. Agamben, *Coming Community*, 1–2.

67. Ibid., 24–25.

68. Ibid., 86.

69. Ben-Levi, "From Euphoria to Sobriety."

70. John Rechy, *City of Night* (New York: Grove Weidenfeld, 1963); Samuel R. Delany, "Appendix A: The Tale of Plagues and Carnivals, or: Some Informal Remarks Toward the Modular Calculus, Part Five," in *Flight from Nevèrÿon* (Hanover, N.H.: Wesleyan University Press / University Press of New England, 1994), 181–359.

71. Ben-Levi, "From Euphoria to Sobriety," 154.

72. Included in Adam Kuby, "The Art of David Wojnarowicz," *Out/Look* 4, no. 4 (Spring 1992): 53–62.

73. Blinderman, *David Wojnarowicz*, 54–56.

74. See Tanizaki Jun'ichirō, *The Secret History of the Lord of Musashi*; and *Arrowroot*, trans. Anthony H. Chambers (New York: Knopf, 1982).

75. Friedrich Nietzsche, "On the Uses and Disadvantages of History for Life," in *Untimely Meditations*, trans. R. J. Hollingdale (Cambridge, Eng.: Cambridge University Press, 1983), 57–123; Michel Foucault, "Nietzsche, Genealogy, History," in *Language, Counter-Memory, Practice: Selected Essays and Interviews*, trans. Donald F. Bouchard and Sherry Simon, ed. Donald F. Bouchard (Ithaca, N.Y.: Cornell University Press, 1977), 139–64.

76. Nietzsche, "Uses and Disadvantages of History," 67–72

77. Foucault, "Nietzsche, Genealogy, History," 160.

78. Ibid., 143.

79. See Alexander Kojève's influential reading of the dialectic of lord and bondsman in *Introduction à la lecture de Hegel*, assembled by Raymond Queneau (Paris: Editions Gallimard, 1947), 10–34.

80. I am indebted to Maureen Turim for suggesting this possibility.

81. Tanizaki Jun'ichirō, *In Praise of Shadows*, trans. Thomas J. Harper and Edward G. Seidensticker (New Haven, Conn.: Leete's Island Books, 1977).

82. The texts by Sue Golding that I have been reading are "The Address Book" (hereafter cited parenthetically in the text as AB), in Paul Hallam, *The Book of Sodom* (London: Verso, 1993), 168–73; "Sexual Manners" (hereafter SM), *Public* 8 (1993): 161–68; "Pariah bodies" (hereafter PB), *Critical Quarterly* 36, no. 1 (Spring 1994): 28–36; "James Dean: The Almost-Perfect Lesbian Hermaphrodite" (hereafter JD), in *Sight Specific: Lesbians and Representation*, ed. Lynne Fernie, Dinah Forbes, and Joyce Mason (Toronto: A Space, 1988), 49–52; "Curiosity" (hereafter C), an unpublished paper presented at Binghamton University, 10 May 1993; and "The Poetics of Foucault's Politics, or, Better Yet: The Ethical Demand of Ecstatic Fetish" (hereafter PFP), in *In Foucault's Wake*, ed. Philip Derbyshire (London: Lawrence & Wishart, forthcoming).

83. One of the best and most succinct psychoanalytic approaches is that

of Jean Laplanche, *Life and Death in Psychoanalysis*, trans. Jeffrey Mehlman (Baltimore: Johns Hopkins University Press, 1976), 85–102.

84. Quoted in David Macey, *The Lives of Michel Foucault* (New York: Pantheon Books, 1993), 365.

85. Ibid., 368–69.

86. See Nishida Kitarō, *Kāteki chokkan no tachiba*, *Kāteki chokkan*, and *Poieshisu to purakushisu*, all in *NKz*, 8: 107–218; 8: 541–71; and 10: 124–76, respectively.

Index

In this index an "f" after a number indicates a separate reference on the next page, and an "ff" indicates separate references on the next two pages. A continuous discussion over two or more pages is indicated by a span of page numbers, e.g., "57–59." *Passim* is used for a cluster of references in close but not consecutive sequence.

Violence: in relation to the erotic, 151–54

Witnessing, *see* Personal testimony
Wojnarowicz, David, xiiff, xvi, 18, 122–59; idea of the predetermined world, 126, 129–32, 134, 138, 181; relation between sex and the erotic in, 132–33; on promiscuity, 142–45; on the funeral, 148–49; the theme of sovereignty in the writings of, 155–56. *See also Close to the Knives*; Ekstases of temporality

Writing: as the limit of experience, 76

Zero-degree aisthesis, 13, 109; in Wojnarowicz, 132; of the lesbian hermaphrodite, 197
Zero-degree historicity, xii
Zero Patience, xii

Library of Congress Cataloging-in-Publication Data

Haver, William Wendell, 1947–
    The body of this death : historicity and sociality in
the time of AIDS / William Haver.
            p.   cm.
    Includes bibliographical references and index.
    ISBN 0-8047-2716-3 (cloth : alk. paper).
    ISBN 0-8047-2728-7 (pbk. : alk. paper)
        1. AIDS (Disease)—Philosophy.   2. AIDS (Disease)—
Social aspects.   I. Title.
RC607.A26H38   1996
306.4´61—dc20   96-856
                                                    CIP

(∞) This book is printed on acid-free paper

Original printing 1996
Last figure below indicates year of this printing
05   04   03   02   01   00   99   98   97   96